HEMATURIA

ETIOLOGY, MANAGEMENT AND LONG-TERM PROGNOSIS

Renal and Urologic Disorders

Additional books in this series can be found on Nova's website
under the Series tab.

Additional e-books in this series can be found on Nova's website
under the e-book tab.

HEMATURIA

ETIOLOGY, MANAGEMENT AND LONG-TERM PROGNOSIS

NIKHIL VASDEV

AND

G. BOUSTEAD

EDITORS

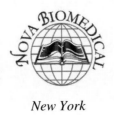

New York

NOTICE TO THE READER

Library of Congress Cataloging-in-Publication Data

ISBN: 978-1-63463-073-3
Library of Congress Control Number: 2014950591

Published by Nova Science Publishers, Inc. † New York

Nikhil Vasdev

To Joanne and Ellie and Eva, who light up and enrich my life.

To Mr. Kailash Vasdev and Mrs. Rita Vasdev, my parent,s and my sister, Neoma, thank you for all your support, for making us what we are and what we stand for.

Gregory Boustead

To Louise, James and Grace

Contents

Preface

Our book titled "Hematuria: Etiology, Management and Long-Term Prognosis" has been complied by a group of doctors and nurses from all the over the world. When we received the honour of being joint editors for this new book, we set our aim to ensure that the reader of our book gets the different perspective of how haematuria is managed all over the world. Chapter contributions have been received from the, UK, USA, Spain, India, Japan, Albania, Singapore and Sri Lanka.

From a patients perspective finding blood in the can be a very frightening experience and must be investigated. Our book helps provides an update on the common Aetiologies and Management of both adult and paediatric patients. In the book there are contributions from both Nephrologist and Urologist discussing the details of both visible and non-visible haematuria which will help guide the reader with the best management strategies for these groups of patients. We also present chapters, which are purely focused on the patients perspective of haematuria.

We hope you enjoy the book.

Mr. Nikhil Vasdev
ChM (Urol), FRCS (Urol)
Consultant Urological and Robotic Surgeon
Hertfordshire and South Bedfordshire Robotic Urological Cancer Centre
Lister Hospital
Stevenage, UK
E-mail – nikhilvasdev@doctors.org.uk

Mr. Gregory Boustead
M. Med (Urol), FRCS (Urol)
Consultant Urological and Robotic Surgeon
Hertfordshire and South Bedfordshire Robotic Urological Cancer Centre
Lister Hospital
Stevenage, UK

17th July 2014

In: Hematuria
Editors: Nikhil Vasdev and G. Boustead

ISBN: 978-1-63463-073-3
© 2015 Nova Science Publishers, Inc.

Chapter 1

Causes and Management of Post Renal Transplant Haematuria

Ho Yee Tiong[*], *BM. BS., MRCS, FAMS*
Department of Urology, National University Hospital
Kidney Surgery and Transplantation
Department of Surgery, Yong Loo Lin School of Medicine, Singapore

Introduction

The kidney transplant population is unique from the general population with its presentation and causes of haematuria. From early reports, its incidences of both microscopic (greater than 4-5 red blood cells per HPF) and gross haematuria have been known to be higher than the general population (up to 12%) [1, 2]. For these patients, evaluation needs to take into consideration traditional urological causes as well as causes from an immunological and nephrological standpoint. As such, the evaluation and treatment of a kidney transplant patient with haematuria may be best served by the urologist working with a multi-disciplinary transplant team.

Urological Causes and Management

Patients with kidney transplantation presenting with haematuria would suffer the same causes – malignancy, stones, and iatrogenic - as the general population. They should therefore undergo the same upper tract and lower tract urological evaluation.

[*] 1E Kent Ridge Road, Singapore 119228. Email: cfsthy@nus.edu.sg; BM. BS. (Hons), MRCS (London), FAMS (Urology). Consultant, Department of Urology, National University Hospital; Director, Kidney Surgery and Transplantation; Assistant Professor, Department of Surgery, Yong Loo Lin School of Medicine

Malignancy

It is widely known that cancers are more common after kidney transplantation than in the general population, and more frequent than in comparable patients on dialysis [3, 4]. The reasons have been attributed to the side effects of immunosuppressive agents, which can cause DNA damage, impair immune surveillance and interfere with normal DNA repair. There is also an increased risk of oncogenic viral infections. With respect to the urinary tract, large scale registry data has shown that urological malignancies are the second or third most common solid organ neoplasm in the renal transplant population.

Prostate cancer is approximately twofold higher in the first 3 years after transplantation than in the general population. Testicular and bladder cancers [5] are increased approximately threefold, while kidney cancer is approximately 15 fold more common. With continually improving outcomes of kidney transplant patients due to advances in immunosuppression, there are increasing advocates to provide screening for prostate cancer [6] and kidney cancer in kidney transplant recipients [7].

In closely screened kidney transplant populations, a high incidence of urinary tract malignancies has been picked up when investigated for haematuria [8, 9]. Hence in renal recipients presenting with haematuria, a careful evaluation of the entire urinary tract for malignancies is crucial.

The management of urological cancers in kidney transplant patients should follow the same protocol as the general population with certain caveats. In localized prostate cancer, experience in radical prostatectomy has been limited but has been shown to be feasible and safe using open, robot-assist or pure laparoscopic approaches [10-12]. Technical modifications are needed to overcome the limited retropubic space occupied by the graft and the need to protect the vascular and uretero-vesical anastomosis. Radiation with androgen deprivation has also been used to treat small series of localized prostate cancer in kidney transplant patients [13, 14]. There is a risk of distal transplant ureteric stricture due to exposure of the vesicoureteric anastomosis in the radiation field. This may be reduced by having a full bladder at the time of irradiation.

The substantial increased risk of renal cancers in the transplant population primarily occurs in the native kidneys, with the known association of cancers with acquired cystic disease of the kidneys [7, 15]. This risk is related to the duration of dialysis before transplant. Treatment is usually straight forward with native radical nephrectomy. As the tumors are often small, they are amenable to laparoscopic treatment [16, 17]. A more difficult problem is the occurrence of cancer in the allograft kidney, with a reported low incidence rate of 0.2-0.4%. Graft nephrectomy is the standard treatment but puts the patient back on dialysis. Partial allograft nephrectomy has been recently attempted via the open and more recently robotic-assisted laparoscopic approach [18, 19].

An important aspect in the immunosuppression regimes of patients after surgical treatment of their urological cancers would be the consideration of conversion of their immunosuppression to one that is Mammalian Target of Rapamycin (MTOR) inhibitor based [20]. Examples of these agents include sirolimus and everolimus. This has been increasingly advocated due to the anti-tumorigenic activity of MTOR inhibitors, especially with respect to kidney cancers [21].

Stones

Stones in native kidneys or the allograft kidney can present with haematuria. Although loin pain or ureteric colic may be a presenting feature of stones in the native kidney and ureter, this may be absent for transplant lithiasis. The latter is more likely to be associated with graft dysfunction or transplant pyelonephritis. Although stones in native failed kidneys or ureter presenting with haematuria can be treated with extracorporeal shockwave lithotripsy (ESWL), larger stones including staghorn stones may be better managed with laparoscopic native nephrectomy. For stones complicating the kidney allograft (reported prevalence of 0.2-6,3%), there is now increasing body of experience of successful treatment using all the available endourological modalities. ESWL has been reported to be successful in clearing kidney transplant stones. Due to the anterior and more superficial location of kidney transplant, considerations for the use of ESWL include use of over the table shockwave delivery or prone patient positioning [22]. There needs to be a reduction in the energy and total number of shocks to decrease the risk of injury to the transplant kidney and a consideration for the use of a temporary nephrostomy tube to provide drainage. Ureteroscopy has also been reported for the treatment of transplant kidney and ureter stones [23]. However, the uretero-vesicalanasotomosis over the bladder dome makes it difficult to pass the scope retrogradely into the transplant ureter and kidney. The surgeon often requires a Klump catheter to do so. Antegrade ureteroscopy can also be utilised if percutaneous renal access is available. Larger transplant kidney stones including staghorn stones and even encrusted forgotten transplant DJ stents will require percutaneous nephrolithotomy [24].

Iatrogenic

It is important to bear in mind that hematuria after kidney transplant is common after the operation itself or after any interventional or diagnostic procedures. Initial gross haematuria after the operation due to mild bleeding from the uretero-cystostomy site is common and self-limiting. A bladder washout may be all that is required to clear the clots and stop bleeding in the early post-operative period. It may be also due to the presence of the DJ stent with associated infection [25] or poor positioning. Hematuria can occur after a kidney transplant biopsy and one should also bear in mind the possibility of pseudo-aneurysm formation after a biopsy [26, 27] or other urological interventions including percutaneous nephrostomy [28] or PCNL. If severe, angioembolization may be needed to stop the bleeding.

Immunological Causes and Management

Urinary Tract Infections

Patients on immunosuppression have increased vulnerability to both common and unique infections. In kidney transplant patients, urinary tract infections are the most common and have been reported to occur at a frequency of between 33 to 54% within the first year of the transplant [29]. These can cause significant morbidity including haematuria as well as transplant pyelonephritis. The bacterial organisms involved are similar to those in the general population including *E. Coli, Klebsiella* and *Pseudomonas* species. The organisms involved also tend to be multi-drug resistant species. As such the optimal treatment is prevention of infection so that the use of potentially nephrotoxic antibiotics can be avoided.. Preventative measures recommended include screening and early treatment for asymptomatic bacteruria in this population [30], early removal of foreign bodies including DJ stents and urethral catheters, as well as routine basic antibiotic prophylaxis during the early transplant phase.

T cell immunosuppression results in increased susceptibility to fungal and viral infections, despite routine prophylaxis. Both cytomegalovirus (CMV) and BK virus have been implicated as causes of microscopic hematuria in transplant patients, with CMV nephritis[2] or BK nephropathy. In significant disease, gross hematuria can occur due to hemorrhagic cystitis [31].

Diagnosis often requires serum detection of CMV or BK viral DNA using PCR and ideally, kidney transplant core needle biopsy under ultrasound guidance is performed to document infection of the transplant. Once proven, treatment of viral infections requires the use of the appropriate anti-viral agents as well as a reduction in the level of immunosuppression [32, 33]. For CMV, the agents used include valganciclovir or ganciclovir. For BK virus, treatment is more complicated and different agents have been tried with limited success, including sirolimus and leflunomide.

Rejections

Acute and chronic rejections of the transplanted kidney can cause haematuria and should be suspected in the presence of graft dysfunction (with an associated rise in baseline creatinine or increase in proteinuria). Diagnosis involves biopsy of the kidney and measurements of donor specific antibodies. Depending on the Banff grade of acute rejection [34] and the type of rejection (cell mediated vs. antibody mediated), treatment options can range from intravenous pulse of steroids, depleting antibody therapy such as thymoglobulin, plasmapheresis to intravenous immunoglobulins [35].

In patients with chronic rejection and a resultant failed kidney transplant, recurrent episodes of gross hematuria are common, especially when the patient has returned to dialysis and immunosuppression has been weaned off. Besides graft failure and gross haematuria, patients will often present with fever in the absence of any infective cause and a painful graft. Examination will confirm a tender and swollen kidney allograft. Urological investigations for the cause of gross haematuria will be negative except for cross sectional imaging findings of a swollen poorly vascularized kidney graft. Transplant nephrectomy is indicated and effective for the treatment of these symptomatic patients with failed graft [36], despite the concerns of increased sensitization after graft nephrectomy [37]. The surgery may carry significant risk of bleeding and some centers have advocated a course of high dose steroids or angio-embolization before graft nephrectomy.

Nephrological Causes and Management

Nephrological causes refer to the native kidney disease or its recurrence in the transplant kidney, resulting in haematuria after kidney transplantation. Autosomal dominant polycystic kidney disease (ADPKD) following kidney transplant is the obvious example and may present with persistent, problematic bleeding, complicated with and without infections [38]. Although the immunosuppression agent MTOR inhibitor such as sirolimus has been reported to be effective in reducing cyst numbers in ADPKD [39], it has not been shown to adequately prevent complications such as haematuria after transplantation. Bilateral or unilateral native nephrectomy can now be performed to treat complications from the large polycystic kidneys. Indeed, simultaneous native nephrectomy and kidney transplantation can be safely performed and is advocated in patients known to have complications from their polycystic disease prior to the transplant [40, 41]. Although laparoscopic cyst decortication can be performed, these are less effective in resolving hematuria from polycystic kidney disease and therefore not ideal.

Certain other disease recurrence can occur in the native or transplant graft kidney. Transplant physicians need to aware of chronic glomerulopathy such as IgA nephropathy and focal segmental glomerulosclerosis (FSGS) which can result in progressive graft failure. Patients often present with graft dysfunction associated with microscopic haematuria and proteinuria. Definitive diagnosis is obtained again with a graft biopsy. Treatment will depend on the underlying condition and require nephrologist input. Although glomerulonephritis of the transplant kidney can be difficult to treat, the treatment options often are the same immunosuppression agents used in kidney transplantation such as steroids, calcineurin inhibitors such as cyclosporine and antimetabolites such as mycophenolatemofetil.

Conclusion

Microscopic and gross haematuria in a kidney transplant patient encompasses the same causes as the normal population as well as unique causes due to the presence of immunosuppression. Treatment is best tailored to each individual patient in the setting of transplant multi-disciplinary team.

References

[1]   Previte, S. R., Murata, G. T., Olsson, C. A. et al.: Hematuria in renal transplant recipients. *Ann. Surg.,* 187: 219, 1978.

[2]   Butani, L., Berg, G., Makker, S. P.: Microhematuria after renal transplantation in children. *Pediatr. Nephrol.,* 17: 1038, 2002.

[3]   Kasiske, B. L., Snyder, J. J., Gilbertson, D. T. et al.: Cancer after kidney transplantation in the United States. *American Journal of Transplantation*, 4: 905, 2004.

[4] Bustami, R. T., Ojo, A. O., Wolfe, R. A. et al.: Immunosuppression and the risk of post-transplant malignancy among cadaveric first kidney transplant recipients. *Am. J. Transplant.*, 4: 87, 2004.

[5] Buzzeo, B. D., Heisey, D. M., Messing, E. M.: Bladder cancer in renal transplant recipients. *Urology*, 50: 525, 1997.

[6] Kiberd, B. A., Keough-Ryan, T., Clase, C. M.: Screening for prostate, breast and colorectal cancer in renal transplant recipients. *Am. J. Transplant.*, 3: 619, 2003.

[7] Goh, A., Vathsala, A.: Native renal cysts and dialysis duration are risk factors for renal cell carcinoma in renal transplant recipients. *Am. J. Transplant.*, 11: 86, 2011.

[8] Kim, D. Y., Abouljoud, M., Parasuraman, R.: The role of microscopic hematuria in the evaluation of urologic malignancy in renal transplant recipients. *Transplant. Proc.*, 42: 1641, 2010.

[9] Tai, H. C., Lai, M. K., Wang, S. M. et al.: High incidence of urinary tract malignancy among patients with haematuria following kidney transplantation in Taiwan. *Transpl. Int.*, 22: 403, 2009.

[10] Smith, D. L., Jellison, F. C., Heldt, J. P. et al.: Robot-assisted radical prostatectomy in patients with previous renal transplantation. *J. Endourol.*, 25: 1643, 2011.

[11] Polcari, A. J., Allen, J. C., Nunez-Nateras, R. et al.: Multicenter experience with robot-assisted radical prostatectomy in renal transplant recipients. *Urology*, 80: 1267, 2012.

[12] Thomas, A. A., Nguyen, M. M., Gill, I. S.: Laparoscopic transperitoneal radical prostatectomy in renal transplant recipients: a review of three cases. *Urology*, 71: 205, 2008.

[13] Binsaleh, S.: Diagnosis and treatment of prostate cancer in renal-transplant recipients. *Int. Urol. Nephrol.*, 44: 149, 2012.

[14] Mouzin, M., Bachaud, J. M., Kamar, N. et al.: Three-dimensional conformal radiotherapy for localized prostate cancer in kidney transplant recipients. *Transplantation*, 78: 1496, 2004.

[15] Schwarz, A., Vatandaslar, S., Merkel, S. et al.: Renal cell carcinoma in transplant recipients with acquired cystic kidney disease. *Clin. J. Am. Soc. Nephrol.*, 2: 750, 2007.

[16] Moudouni, S. M., Lakmichi, A., Tligui, M. et al.: Renal cell carcinoma of native kidney in renal transplant recipients. *BJU Int.*, 98: 298, 2006.

[17] Ianhez, L. E., Lucon, M., Nahas, W. C. et al.: Renal cell carcinoma in renal transplant patients. *Urology*, 69: 462, 2007.

[18] Kaouk, J. H., Spana, G., Hillyer, S. P. et al.: Robotic-Assisted Laparoscopic Partial Nephrectomy for a 7-cm Mass in a Renal Allograft. *American Journal of Transplantation*, 11: 2242, 2011.

[19] Barama, A., St-Louis, G., Nicolet, V. et al.: Renal cell carcinoma in kidney allografts: a case series from a single center. *Am. J. Transplant.*, 5: 3015, 2005.

[20] Chiurchiu, C., Carreno, C. A., Schiavelli, R. et al.: Results of the conversion to everolimus in renal transplant recipients with posttransplantation malignancies. *Transplant. Proc.*, 42: 277, 2010.

[21] Hudes, G., Carducci, M., Tomczak, P. et al.: Temsirolimus, interferon alfa, or both for advanced renal-cell carcinoma. *The New England journal of medicine*, 356: 2271, 2007.

[22] Wheatley, M., Ohl, D. A., Sonda, L. P., 3rd et al.: Treatment of renal transplant stones by extracorporeal shock-wave lithotripsy in the prone position. *Urology*, 37: 57, 1991.

[23] Hyams, E., Marien, T., Bruhn, A. et al.: Ureteroscopy for transplant lithiasis. *J. Endourol.*, 26: 819, 2012.

[24] Romanowsky, I., Lupu, L., Lismer, L. et al.: Percutaneous nephrolithotomy in transplanted kidney--forgotten stent with complete staghorn and large bladder stone. Case report. *Transpl. Int.*, 17: 877, 2005.

[25] Glazier, D. B., Jacobs, M. G., Lyman, N. W. et al.: Urinary tract infection associated with ureteral stents in renal transplantation. *Can. J. Urol.*, 5: 462, 1998.

[26] Furness, P. N., Philpott, C. M., Chorbadjian, M. T. et al.: Protocol biopsy of the stable renal transplant: a multicenter study of methods and complication rates. *Transplantation*, 76: 969, 2003.

[27] Voiculescu, A., Brause, M., Engelbrecht, V. et al.: Hemodynamically relevant hematuria several months after biopsy of a kidney graft: an unusual cause. *Clin. Nephrol.*, 59: 217, 2003.

[28] Ladinsky, G. A., Goral, S.: Macroscopic hematuria in a kidney transplant recipient: a rare cause. *Am. J. Kidney Dis.*, 47: e3, 2006.

[29] Rivera-Sanchez, R., Delgado-Ochoa, D., Flores-Paz, R. R. et al.: Prospective study of urinary tract infection surveillance after kidney transplantation. *BMC Infect. Dis.*, 10: 245, 2010.

[30] Fiorante, S., Lopez-Medrano, F., Lizasoain, M. et al.: Systematic screening and treatment of asymptomatic bacteriuria in renal transplant recipients. *Kidney Int.*, 78: 774, 2010.

[31] Singh, D., Kiberd, B., Gupta, R. et al.: Polyoma virus-induced hemorrhagic cystitis in renal transplantation patient with polyoma virus nephropathy. *Urology*, 67: 423 e11, 2006.

[32] Hodson, E., Craig, J., Strippoli, G. et al.: Antiviral medications for preventing cytomegalovirus disease in solid organ transplant recipients. *Cochrane database of systematic reviews* (Online), (2): CD003774, 2008.

[33] Bohl, D. L., Brennan, D. C.: BK virus nephropathy and kidney transplantation. *Clin. J. Am. Soc. Nephrol.*, 2 Suppl 1: S36, 2007.

[34] Racusen, L. C., Solez, K., Colvin, R. B. et al.: The Banff 97 working classification of renal allograft pathology. *Kidney Int.*, 55: 713, 1999.

[35] Halloran, P. F.: Immunosuppressive drugs for kidney transplantation. *N. Engl. J. Med.*, 351: 2715, 2004.

[36] Evans, D. H., Luger, A. M., Ross, G., Jr. et al.: Gross hematuria requiring nephrectomy in rejected renal transplants. *J. Urol.*, 128: 125, 1982.

[37] Knight, M. G., Tiong, H. Y., Li, J. et al.: Transplant nephrectomy after allograft failure is associated with allosensitization. *Urology*, 78: 314, 2011.

[38] Torres, V. E., Harris, P. C., Pirson, Y.: Autosomal dominant polycystic kidney disease. *Lancet*, 369: 1287, 2007.

[39] Qian, Q., Du, H., King, B. F. et al.: Sirolimus reduces polycystic liver volume in ADPKD patients. *Journal of the American Society of Nephrology*, 19: 631, 2008.

[40] Kramer, A., Sausville, J., Haririan, A. et al.: Simultaneous bilateral native nephrectomy and living donor renal transplantation are successful for polycystic kidney disease: the University of Maryland experience. *J. Urol.*, 181: 724, 2009.

[41] Wu, F., Deng, Z., Consigliere, D. et al.: Synchronous nephrectomy with unilateral dual kidney transplantation: feasibility in patients with adult polycystic kidney disease. *Singapore Med. J.,* 53: e163, 2012.

In: Hematuria
Editors: Nikhil Vasdev and G. Boustead

ISBN: 978-1-63463-073-3
© 2015 Nova Science Publishers, Inc.

Chapter 2

Haemorrhagic Cystitis by BK Virus in Haematopoietic Stem Cell Transplantation

Christian Harkensee, M.D., Ph.D., FRCPCH*

Paediatric Immunology, Infectious Diseases & Allergy
Division of Paediatric Infectious Diseases, Department of Paediatrics
National University Hospital Singapore, Singapore

Background

Haemorrhagic cystitis (HC), characterised by haemorrhagic inflammation of the bladder mucosa leading to painful micturation with haematuria, is a rare but severe complication of haematopoietic stem cell transplantation (HSCT). Clinically HC can be mild and brief (Grade I), ranging to severe, prolonged and life-threatening (Grade IV) [1, 2] (table 1).

Table I. Clinical grading of HC [75]

Grade	Clinical Features
I	Microscopic haematuria
II	Macroscopic haematuria
III	Macroscopic haematuria with blood clots
IV	Macroscopic haematuria, blood clots, urinary obstruction, renal impairment, bladder impairment

Whereas early-onset HC (within days after transplantation) is usually mild, self-limiting and associated with the conditioning regimen; late-onset, post-engraftment disease is

* Email: christian_harkensee@nuhs.edu.sg. Consultant in Paediatric Immunology; Assistant Professor in Paediatrics.

associated with the reactivation of urotropic viruses (BK virus [BKV], Adenovirus and Cytomegalyvirus [CMV]) [3]. BK virus infection constitutes between 50-80% of all late-onset HC in HSCT in children.

Late onset HC could be regarded as 'engraftment disease', with onset usually within a month of neutrophil engraftment, followed by variable disease severity and duration (1 week to 4 months) [4]. This variability suggests multiple contributing risk factors, such as pre-transplant viral status, conditioning and immunosuppressive regimens, degree of cellular immunosuppression, Graft-versus-Host Disease (GvHD) and host/donor genetics. Leung et al. [5] have suggested a 3-phase model for post-engraftment HC: uroepithelial insult by chemotherapy and radiation providing a permissive environment for virus replication (phase 1), which is reactivated in the face of immunosuppression (phase 2). Upon engraftment, infected uroepithelial cells are attacked by donor lymphoid cells, leading to tissue destruction (phase 3).

BK Virus. BK virus is a double-stranded DNA virus and was first described in 1971, isolated in cell culture from the urine of an asymptomatic immunosuppressed patient [6]. BKV infection is ubiquitous [7], primary infection with BKV usually occurs in childhood and is generally asymptomatic. Thereafter the virus lies latent in the host, although 5-10% of seropositive individuals shed the virus in the urine asymptomatically at any given time [7]. BKV is urotheliotropic, affecting epithelia of renal calyces, renal pelvis, ureter and urinary bladder. The widespread frequency of BK virus in children suggests common routes of transmission such as respiratory or faecal-oral spread. Nosocomial transmission in HSCT patients has been described [8], therefore appropriate infection control measures are important.

Diagnosis and Risk Factors for BKV Infection in HSCT

BK virus infection during HSCT is largely due to reactivation of dormant virus, although new infection and transmission has also been postulated [5, 9-11].

Urinary BK viral load peaks correlate with subsequent development of HC [5, 12-14]. Up to 50% of HSCT patients have a degree of viruria, although <20% develop HC, requiring the establishment of cut-off viral load values for predicting HC which are still controversial. Blood viral titres $>10^4$ copies/ml preceded onset of HC by a median of 10 days [15, 16]. A urine BK virus load of $>9 \times 10^6$, and blood BKV load $>1 \times 10^3$ copies was predictive of HC in children, with a higher sensitivity for urine monitoring [17]. Viruria preceded onset of clinical HC by a median of 18 days, viraemia by 17 days. Plasma viral loads may predict better severity of renal complications (renal dysfunction, severity of HC, need for dialysis [18, 19] and resolution of HC [20].

Incidence is varied across different transplant populations, ranging from 3.6% to 20%, using different definitions for HC. A number of prospective and retrospective case series have investigated risk factors for the development of post-engraftment HC: myeloablative conditioning [21], unrelated donor transplants [22-24], peripheral blood stem cell transplant [25, 26] and Adenovirus and CMV infection [27-30]. Demographic risk features include male sex [29, 31] and late childhood age range (age >5y/>10 years) [32-35]. GvHD is a consistent risk factor in paediatric [31, 35, 36] mixed [34, 37, 38] and adult [24] study cohorts. Busulphan [23, 33] and cyclophosphamide conditioning [35, 39] and pelvic radiotherapy [26], important risk factors for pre-engraftment HC, seem to also increase risk of post-engraftment HC. Immunosuppressive therapies, including T-cell depletion, ATG, methotrexate, alemtuzumab, cyclosporin and tacrolimus all lead to a higher incidence of HC [23, 31, 40-42]. Newer research did not find busulphan, ATG and cyclophosphamide to be associated with a higher risk for HC unless used in a myeloablative regimen [25].

Management

While pre-engraftment appears to be closely related to the toxic insult of the conditioning regimen, post-engraftment HC is an interplay between BK virus and a local inflammatory environment, cellular immune responses, effector mechanisms, and HLA as well as non-HLA genetics. Any measures that reduce the toxic insult of conditioning, prevent GvHD, limit immunosuppression, and promote rapid and functional engraftment will impact on incidence and severity of post-engraftment HC.

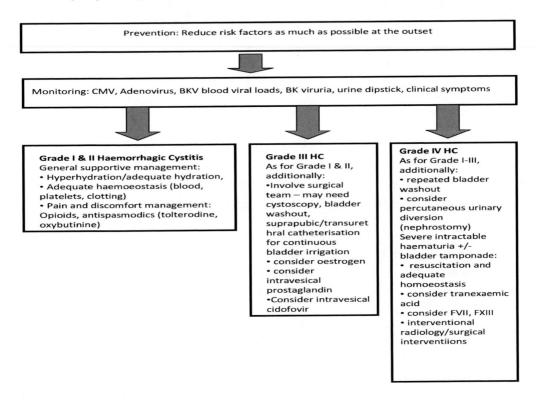

Figure 1. Management of HC.

The management of the child with HC is difficult. The condition is potentially life threatening and causing extensive discomfort. Conditioning, profound immunosuppression and co-morbidities such as renal impairment restrict therapeutic options. The approach to the patient with HC encompasses:

- Prevention by addressing known risk factors early: best possible donor-recipient matching, using the least toxic conditioning regimen possible with MESNA/hyperhydration, tight monitoring of viral titres (CMV, Adenovirus) and prompt treatment of re-activation in the peri-transplant period, GvHD prevention and tightly monitored immunosuppression.

- Optimal supportive treatment of manifest HC: ensuring appropriate hydration and renal function, haematological homoeostasis, pain relief, catheterisation with cystoscopic clot extraction and continuous bladder irrigation, if necessary.

- Early and close collaboration between medical and surgical teams in the management of these patients to coordinate and optimise timing of interventions.

- As post-engraftment HC is by nature a transient condition that resolves with immune reconstitution – a 'conservative' approach avoiding measures that may inflict long-term consequences on the patient is warranted. Any further interventions would have to be considered on an individual basis for a given clinical scenario, carefully balancing benefits and risks.

The management of HC and treatment options has been subject of a systematic review [43] and is summarized in figure 1.

Medical Treatment Options

Cidofovir has the highest known specificity against BKV although significant nephrotoxicity limits routine use following HSCT where patients are usually concomitantly exposed to other nephrotoxic drugs. High dose (5mg/kg) or low dose (1mg/kg) iv cidofovir resulted in clinical improvement, but not microbial resolution [44, 45]. In a recent retrospective study from Europe, cidofovir lead to reduction in BKV load and clinical improvement (84%), however, about one third of patients had nephrotoxic side effects [46]. The combination with probenecid could potentially reduce the risk of nephrotoxicity [47].

More recently, case reports [48, 49] describe intravesical administration of cidofovir as an alternative to systemic therapy, leading to clinical improvement and reduction of viruria.

Oestrogen. Oestrogen has anti-inflammatory properties, and doses of 25-100 mg/d of iv oestrogen, followed by oral doses of 5-10 mg/d have been used in the treatment of HC with some effect [35, 50, 51]. Side effects are rare, although cases of hepatosis requiring treatment withdrawal have been reported [51].

Hyperbaric Oxygen. Hyperbaric oxygen therapy (HOT), through an increased oxygen pressure in tissues and stimulation of neovascularisation, has a healing effect on necrotic or injured tissues. Although relatively non-toxic, its use has limitations due to the availability of decompression chambers and suitability for sick patients. A number of cases and series report clinical remission in up to 78% of cases [32, 52, 53].

Clotting factors, such as Recombinant activated Factor VII [54, 55, 56] and Factor XIII [57, 58] have been used in HC for their haemostatic and wound healing effects. Factor VII has proven efficacy in stopping severe bleeding in a randomized controlled trial which involves children with HC, but treatment lead to 6% of thromboembolic complications and 2% of deaths.

Keratinocyte growth factor. Anecdotal cases of improvement of HC with Keratinocyte growth factor have been reported [59].

Intravesical prostaglandin instillation. On bladder mucosa, prostaglandin is thought to encourage platelet aggregation and cause contraction of vascular smooth muscle. Prostaglandin is as effective, but less toxic than alum salts [60]. Vesical spasm as a side effect are common but can be controlled with antispasmodics. Instillation of either 0.75 mg/d of PGE2 [61], 500µg/d [62] or 375µg/d of PGE1 [63], or 0.4-1.0mg of intravesical carboprost tromethamine four times/day have been used. A dose of 0.8 mg/dl/h appeared to be a cut-off for a minimum effective dose in continuous irrigation [64].

Intravesical alum salt instillation. Alum salts, administered as a 0.5-1% solution by continuous bladder irrigation, precipitate surface proteins, decrease capillary permeability, and lead subsequently to a reduction in inflammation, oedema and exsudates [65]. Alum salts are affordable and therefore commonly used but are potentially toxic, resulting in encephalopathy and even death, especially in the context of renal impairment, making alum salts a drug to be used with caution.

Intravesical formalin instillation. On the mucosal bladder, formalin precipitates proteins, and occludes and fixates teleangiectatic tissue. Formalin is effective and cheap, however, has a relatively high rate of side effects and complications. Administration is painful and requires regional or general anaesthesia. Complications such as irreversible bladder fibrosis, renal failure, bladder perforation or systemic toxicity are common. A drug escalation study [66], administering 1%, 2% and 4% formalin in three different arms, demonstrated no significant difference in the response rate. The higher concentrations of formalin, however, lead to an increased risk of major complications, which were 31% overall.

Intravesical instillation of growth factors. A number of cases have been reported successful treatment of intractable HC with intravesical irrigation of recombinant growth factors (G-CSF [67], EGF [68]). Newer approaches include adoptive immunotherapy with BKV specific T-cells is in the experimental stage [69]. Leflunamide is a immunosuppressive agent with antiviral properties against BKV. A small case series [70] describes efficacy in reducing viral load, but no clinical trials have been conducted so far.

Surgical Treatment Options

Cystoscopic cauterization and application of fibrin glue has been described in a case report [71]. *Selective Embolization* by retrograde catheterization of the vesical artery has been applied in single case [72]. *Intravesical Hydrostatic Pressure* applied with a balloon is a temporary measure to achieve haemostasis [73]. *Cystectomy* is seen as the ultima ratio to stop bleeding in intractable HC [74].

References

[1]   Bedi A, Miller CB, Hanson JL, Goodman S, Ambinder RF, Charache P, et al., Association of BK virus with failure of prophylaxis against hemorrhagic cystitis following bone marrow transplantation. *J. Clin. Oncol.* 1995;13(5):1103-9.

[2]   Iwamoto S, Azuma E, Hori H, Hirayama M, Kobayashi M, Komada Y, et al., BK virus-associated fatal renal failure following late-onset hemorrhagic cystitis in an unrelated bone marrow transplantation. *Pediatr. Hematol. Oncol.* 2002;19(4):255-61.

[3]   Leung AY, Mak R, Lie AK, Yuen KY, Cheng VC, Liang R, et al., Clinicopathological features and risk factors of clinically overt haemorrhagic cystitis complicating bone marrow transplantation. *Bone Marrow Transplant* 2002;29(6):509-13.

[4]   McCarville MB, Hoffer FA, Gingrich JR, Jenkins JJ, 3rd. Imaging findings of hemorrhagic cystitis in pediatric oncology patients. *Pediatr Radiol.* 2000;30(3):131-8.

[5]   Leung AY, Chan MT, Yuen KY, Cheng VC, Chan KH, Wong CL, et al., Ciprofloxacin decreased polyoma BK virus load in patients who underwent allogeneic hematopoietic stem cell transplantation. *Clin. Infect Dis.* 2005;40(4):528-37.

[6]   Gardner SD, Field AM, Coleman DV, Hulme B. New human papovavirus (B.K.) isolated from urine after renal transplantation. *Lancet* 1971;1(7712):1253-7.

[7]   Egli A, Infanti L, Dumoulin A, Buser A, Samaridis J, Stebler C, et al., Prevalence of polyomavirus BK and JC infection and replication in 400 healthy blood donors. *J. Infect Dis.* 2009;199(6):837-46.

[8]   Koskenvuo M, Dumoulin A, Lautenschlager I, Auvinen E, Mannonen L, Anttila VJ, et al., BK polyomavirus-associated hemorrhagic cystitis among pediatric allogeneic bone marrow transplant recipients: treatment response and evidence for nosocomial transmission. *J. Clin. Virol.* 2013;56(1):77-81.

[9]   Bohl DL, Storch GA, Ryschkewitsch C, Gaudreault-Keener M, Schnitzler MA, Major EO, et al., Donor origin of BK virus in renal transplantation and role of HLA C7 in susceptibility to sustained BK viremia. *Am. J. Transplant* 2005;5(9):2213-21.

[10]   Bogdanovic G, Priftakis P, Taemmeraes B, Gustafsson A, Flaegstad T, Winiarski J, et al., Primary BK virus (BKV) infection due to possible BKV transmission during bone marrow transplantation is not the major cause of hemorrhagic cystitis in transplanted children. *Pediatr Transplant* 1998;2(4):288-93.

[11]   Dolei A, Pietropaolo V, Gomes E, Di Taranto C, Ziccheddu M, Spanu MA, et al., Polyomavirus persistence in lymphocytes: prevalence in lymphocytes from blood donors and healthy personnel of a blood transfusion centre. *J. Gen. Virol.* 2000;81(Pt 8):1967-73.

[12]   Azzi A, Cesaro S, Laszlo D, Zakrzewska K, Ciappi S, De Santis R, et al., Human polyomavirus BK (BKV) load and haemorrhagic cystitis in bone marrow transplantation patients. *J. Clin. Virol.* 1999;14(2):79-86.

[13]   Leung AY, Suen CK, Lie AK, Liang RH, Yuen KY, Kwong YL. Quantification of polyoma BK viruria in hemorrhagic cystitis complicating bone marrow transplantation. *Blood* 2001;98(6):1971-8.

[14]   Bogdanovic G, Priftakis P, Giraud G, Kuzniar M, Ferraldeschi R, Kokhaei P, et al., Association between a high BK virus load in urine samples of patients with graft-versus-host disease and development of hemorrhagic cystitis after hematopoietic stem cell transplantation. *J. Clin. Microbiol.* 2004;42(11):5394-6.

[15]   Erard V, Kim HW, Corey L, Limaye A, Huang ML, Myerson D, et al., BK DNA viral load in plasma: evidence for an association with hemorrhagic cystitis in allogeneic hematopoietic cell transplant recipients. *Blood* 2005;106(3):1130-2.

[16]   Erard V, Storer B, Corey L, Nollkamper J, Huang ML, Limaye A, et al., BK virus infection in hematopoietic stem cell transplant recipients: frequency, risk factors, and

association with postengraftment hemorrhagic cystitis. *Clin. Infect Dis.* 2004;39(12):1861-5.

[17]   Cesaro S, Facchin C, Tridello G, Messina C, Calore E, Biasolo MA, et al., A prospective study of BK-virus-associated haemorrhagic cystitis in paediatric patients undergoing allogeneic haematopoietic stem cell transplantation. *Bone Marrow Transplant* 2007.

[18]   Haines HL, Laskin BL, Goebel J, Davies SM, Yin HJ, Lawrence J, et al., Blood, and not urine, BK viral load predicts renal outcome in children with hemorrhagic cystitis following hematopoietic stem cell transplantation. *Biol. Blood Marrow Transplant* 2011;17(10):1512-9.

[19]   Oshrine B, Bunin N, Li Y, Furth S, Laskin BL. Kidney and bladder outcomes in children with hemorrhagic cystitis and BK virus infection after allogeneic hematopoietic stem cell transplantation. *Biol. Blood Marrow Transplant* 2013;19(12):1702-7.

[20]   Drew RJ, Walsh A, Ni Laoi B, Conneally E, Crowley B. BK virus (BKV) plasma dynamics in patients with BKV-associated hemorrhagic cystitis following allogeneic stem cell transplantation. *Transpl. Infect Dis.* 2013;15(3):276-82.

[21]   Giraud G, Bogdanovic G, Priftakis P, Remberger M, Svahn BM, Barkholt L, et al., The incidence of hemorrhagic cystitis and BK-viruria in allogeneic hematopoietic stem cell recipients according to intensity of the conditioning regimen. *Haematologica* 2006;91(3):401-4.

[22]   Bogdanovic G, Priftakis P, Giraud G, Dalianis T. A related donor and reduced intensity conditioning reduces the risk of development of BK virus-positive haemorrhagic cystitis in allogeneic haematopoetic stem cell-transplanted patients. *Anticancer Res* 2006;26(2B):1311-8.

[23]   Trotman J, Nivison-Smith I, Dodds A. Haemorrhagic cystitis: incidence and risk factors in a transplant population using hyperhydration. *Bone Marrow Transplant* 1999;23(8):797-801.

[24]   Chakrabarti S, Osman H, Collingham K, Milligan DW. Polyoma viruria following T-cell-depleted allogeneic transplants using Campath-1H: incidence and outcome in relation to graft manipulation, donor type and conditioning. *Bone Marrow Transplant* 2003;31(5):379-86.

[25]   Anoop P, Shaw BE, Riley U, Ethell ME, Taj M, Lancaster DL, et al., Clinical profile and outcome of urotheliotropic viral haemorrhagic cystitis following haematopoietic stem cell transplantation: a 7-year tertiary centre analysis. *Hematology* 2011;16(4):213-20.

[26]   Riachy E, Krauel L, Rich BS, McEvoy MP, Honeyman JN, Boulad F, et al., Risk factors and predictors of severity score and complications of pediatric hemorrhagic cystitis. *J. Urol.* 2014;191(1):186-92.

[27]   Yamamoto R, Kusumi E, Kami M, Yuji K, Hamaki T, Saito A, et al., Late hemorrhagic cystitis after reduced-intensity hematopoietic stem cell transplantation (RIST). *Bone Marrow Transplant* 2003;32(11):1089-95.

[28]   Akiyama H, Kurosu T, Sakashita C, Inoue T, Mori S, Ohashi K, et al., Adenovirus is a key pathogen in hemorrhagic cystitis associated with bone marrow transplantation. *Clin. Infect Dis.* 2001;32(9):1325-30.

[29] Asano Y, Kanda Y, Ogawa N, Sakata-Yanagimoto M, Nakagawa M, Kawazu M, et al., Male predominance among Japanese adult patients with late-onset hemorrhagic cystitis after hematopoietic stem cell transplantation. *Bone Marrow Transplant* 2003;32(12):1175-9.

[30] Tomonari A, Takahashi S, Ooi J, Fukuno K, Takasugi K, Tsukada N, et al., Hemorrhagic cystitis in adults after unrelated cord blood transplantation: a single-institution experience in Japan. *Int. J. Hematol.* 2006;84(3):268-71.

[31] Hale GA, Rochester RJ, Heslop HE, Krance RA, Gingrich JR, Benaim E, et al., Hemorrhagic cystitis after allogeneic bone marrow transplantation in children: clinical characteristics and outcome. *Biol. Blood Marrow Transplant* 2003;9(11):698-705.

[32] Cesaro S, Brugiolo A, Faraci M, Uderzo C, Rondelli R, Favre C, et al., Incidence and treatment of hemorrhagic cystitis in children given hematopoietic stem cell transplantation: a survey from the Italian association of pediatric hematology oncology-bone marrow transplantation group. *Bone Marrow Transplant* 2003;32(9):925-31.

[33] Kondo M, Kojima S, Kato K, Matsuyama T. Late-onset hemorrhagic cystitis after hematopoietic stem cell transplantation in children. *Bone Marrow Transplant* 1998;22(10):995-8.

[34] Seber A, Shu XO, Defor T, Sencer S, Ramsay N. Risk factors for severe hemorrhagic cystitis following BMT. *Bone Marrow Transplant* 1999;23(1):35-40.

[35] Cheuk DK, Lee TL, Chiang AK, Ha SY, Lau YL, Chan GC. Risk factors and treatment of hemorrhagic cystitis in children who underwent hematopoietic stem cell transplantation. *Transpl. Int.* 2007;20(1):73-81.

[36] Russell SJ, Vowels MR, Vale T. Haemorrhagic cystitis in paediatric bone marrow transplant patients: an association with infective agents, GVHD and prior cyclophosphamide. *Bone Marrow Transplant* 1994;13(5):533-9.

[37] El-Zimaity M, Saliba R, Chan K, Shahjahan M, Carrasco A, Khorshid O, et al., Hemorrhagic cystitis after allogeneic hematopoietic stem cell transplantation: donor type matters. *Blood* 2004;103(12):4674-80.

[38] Hassan Z, Remberger M, Svenberg P, Elbander M, Omazic B, Mattsson J, et al., Hemorrhagic cystitis: a retrospective single-center survey. *Clin. Transplant* 2007;21(5):659-67.

[39] Brugieres L, Hartmann O, Travagli JP, Benhamou E, Pico JL, Valteau D, et al., Hemorrhagic cystitis following high-dose chemotherapy and bone marrow transplantation in children with malignancies: incidence, clinical course, and outcome. *J. Clin. Oncol.* 1989;7(2):194-9.

[40] Childs R, Sanchez C, Engler H, Preuss J, Rosenfeld S, Dunbar C, et al., High incidence of adeno- and polyomavirus-induced hemorrhagic cystitis in bone marrow allotransplantation for hematological malignancy following T cell depletion and cyclosporine. *Bone Marrow Transplant* 1998;22(9):889-93.

[41] Agha I, Brennan DC. BK virus and immunosuppressive agents. *Adv. Exp. Med. Biol.* 2006;577:174-84.

[42] Wu C, Randhawa P, McCauley J. Transplantation: polyomavirus nephropathy and the risk of specific immunosuppression regimens. *ScientificWorldJournal* 2006:512-28.

[43] Harkensee C, Vasdev N, Gennery AR, Willetts IE, Taylor C. Prevention and management of BK-virus associated haemorrhagic cystitis in children following

haematopoietic stem cell transplantation--a systematic review and evidence-based guidance for clinical management. *Br. J. Haematol.* 2008;142(5):717-31.

[44] Gorczynska E, Turkiewicz D, Rybka K, Toporski J, Kalwak K, Dyla A, et al., Incidence, clinical outcome, and management of virus-induced hemorrhagic cystitis in children and adolescents after allogeneic hematopoietic cell transplantation. *Biol. Blood Marrow Transplant* 2005;11(10):797-804.

[45] Savona MR, Newton D, Frame D, Levine JE, Mineishi S, Kaul DR. Low-dose cidofovir treatment of BK virus-associated hemorrhagic cystitis in recipients of hematopoietic stem cell transplant. *Bone Marrow Transplant* 2007;39(12):783-7.

[46] Cesaro S, Pillon M, Tridello G, Aljurf M, Martino R, Schroyens W, et al., Relationship between clinical and BK virological response in patients with late hemorrhagic cystitis treated with cidofovir: a retrospective study from the European Group for Blood and Marrow Transplantation. *Bone Marrow Transplant* 2013;48(6):809-13.

[47] Kwon HJ, Kang JH, Lee JW, Chung NG, Kim HK, Cho B. Treatment of BK virus-associated hemorrhagic cystitis in pediatric hematopoietic stem cell transplant recipients with cidofovir: a single-center experience. *Transpl. Infect Dis.* 2013;15(6):569-74.

[48] Walden O, Haertel, C., Doehn, C., Jocham, C. Intravesikale Cidofovir-Instillationstherapie bei Polyomavirus-assoziierter haemorrhagischer Zystitis nach Knochenmarktransplantation. *Der. Urologe* 2006.

[49] Bridges B, Donegan S, Badros A. Cidofovir bladder instillation for the treatment of BK hemorrhagic cystitis after allogeneic stem cell transplantation. *Am. J. Hematol.* 2006;81(7):535-7.

[50] Heath JA, Mishra S, Mitchell S, Waters KD, Tiedemann K. Estrogen as treatment of hemorrhagic cystitis in children and adolescents undergoing bone marrow transplantation. *Bone Marrow Transplant* 2006;37(5):523-6.

[51] Ordemann R, Naumann R, Geissler G, Bornhauser M, Schuler U, Ehninger G. Encouraging results in the treatment of haemorrhagic cystitis with estrogen - report of 10 cases and review of the literature. *Bone Marrow Transplant* 2000;25(9):981-5.

[52] Hattori K, Yabe M, Matsumoto M, Kudo Y, Yasuda Y, Inoue H, et al., Successful hyperbaric oxygen treatment of life-threatening hemorrhagic cystitis after allogeneic bone marrow transplantation. *Bone Marrow Transplant* 2001;27(12):1315-7.

[53] Furness PD, 3rd, Palmer LS, Palmer JS, Capelli-Schellpfeffer M, Cheng EY. Hyperbaric oxygen therapy for pediatric hemorrhagic cystitis. *J. Urol.* 1999;161(5):1596-7.

[54] Pihusch M, Bacigalupo A, Szer J, von Depka Prondzinski M, Gaspar-Blaudschun B, Hyveled L, et al., Recombinant activated factor VII in treatment of bleeding complications following hematopoietic stem cell transplantation. *J. Thromb. Haemost.* 2005;3(9):1935-44.

[55] Ashrani AA, Gabriel DA, Gajewski JL, Jacobs DR, Jr., Weisdorf DJ, Key NS. Pilot study to test the efficacy and safety of activated recombinant factor VII (NovoSeven) in the treatment of refractory hemorrhagic cystitis following high-dose chemotherapy. *Bone Marrow Transplant* 2006;38(12):825-8.

[56] Blatt J, Gold SH, Wiley JM, Monahan PE, Cooper HC, Harvey D. Off-label use of recombinant factor VIIa in patients following bone marrow transplantation. *Bone Marrow Transplant* 2001;28(4):405-7.

[57] Sakuma H, Satoh T, Matsumoto E, Kanno H, Watanabe M, Kikuta A, et al. [The clinical effect of factor XIII on drug-induced hemorrhagic cystitis]. *Rinsho Ketsueki* 1994;35(3):279-85.

[58] Demesmay K, Tissot E, Bulabois CE, Bertrand MA, Racadot E, Woronoff-Lemsi MC, et al., Factor XIII replacement in stem-cell transplant recipients with severe hemorrhagic cystitis: a report of four cases. *Transplantation* 2002;74(8):1190-2.

[59] Czibere A, Bruns I, Graef T, Fenk R, Zohren F, Safaian N, et al., Treatment of severe hemorrhagic cystitis after allogeneic stem cell transplantation with palifermin, a recombinant human keratinocyte growth factor. *Biol. Blood Marrow Transplant* 2007;13(7):872-4.

[60] Praveen BV, Sankaranarayanan A, Vaidyanathan S. A comparative study of intravesical instillation of 15(s) 15 Me alpha and alum in the management of persistent hematuria of vesical origin. *Int. J. Clin. Pharmacol. Ther. Toxicol.* 1992;30(1):7-12.

[61] Laszlo D, Bosi A, Guidi S, Saccardi R, Vannucchi AM, Lombardini L, et al., Prostaglandin E2 bladder instillation for the treatment of hemorrhagic cystitis after allogeneic bone marrow transplantation. *Haematologica* 1995;80(5):421-5.

[62] Nakaseko C, Oh H, Sato H, Cho R, Ishii A, Ikegami T, et al. [Prostaglandin E1 bladder instillations for late-onset hemorrhagic cystitis following allogeneic bone marrow transplantation]. *Rinsho Ketsueki* 1995;36(8):728-34.

[63] Trigg ME, O'Reilly J, Rumelhart S, Morgan D, Holida M, de Alarcon P. Prostaglandin E1 bladder instillations to control severe hemorrhagic cystitis. *J. Urol.* 1990;143(1):92-4.

[64] Ippoliti C, Przepiorka D, Mehra R, Neumann J, Wood J, Claxton D, et al., Intravesicular carboprost for the treatment of hemorrhagic cystitis after marrow transplantation. *Urology* 1995;46(6):811-5.

[65] Arrizabalaga M, Extramiana J, Parra JL, Ramos C, Diaz Gonzalez R, Leiva O. Treatment of massive haematuria with aluminous salts. *Br. J. Urol.* 1987;60(3):223-6.

[66] Dewan AK, Mohan GM, Ravi R. Intravesical formalin for hemorrhagic cystitis following irradiation of cancer of the cervix. *Int. J. Gynaecol. Obstet* 1993;42(2):131-5.

[67] Vela-Ojeda J, Tripp-Villanueva F, Sanchez-Cortes E, Ayala-Sanchez M, Garcia-Ruiz Esparza MA, Rosas-Cabral A, et al., Intravesical rhGM-CSF for the treatment of late onset hemorrhagic cystitis after bone marrow transplant. *Bone Marrow Transplant* 1999;24(12):1307-10.

[68] Dorticos E, Pavon V, Jaime JC, Reboredo M, Lopez Saura P, Berlanga J, et al., Successful application of epidermal growth factor for treatment of hemorrhagic cystitis after bone marrow transplantation. *Bone Marrow Transplant* 2003;31(7):615-6.

[69] Blyth E, Clancy L, Simms R, Gaundar S, O'Connell P, Micklethwaite K, et al., BK virus-specific T cells for use in cellular therapy show specificity to multiple antigens and polyfunctional cytokine responses. *Transplantation* 2011;92(10):1077-84.

[70] Chen XC, Liu T, Li JJ, He C, Meng WT, Huang R. Efficacy and safety of leflunomide for the treatment of BK virus-associated hemorrhagic cystitis in allogeneic hematopoietic stem cell transplantation recipients. *Acta Haematol.* 2013;130(1):52-6.

[71] Purves JT, Graham ML, Ramakumar S. Application of fibrin glue to damaged bladder mucosa in a case of BK viral hemorrhagic cystitis. *Urology* 2005;66(3):641-3.

[72] Gine E, Rovira M, Real I, Burrel M, Montana J, Carreras E, et al., Successful treatment of severe hemorrhagic cystitis after hemopoietic cell transplantation by selective embolization of the vesical arteries. *Bone Marrow Transplant* 2003;31(10):923-5.

[73] Helmstein K. Treatment of bladder carcinoma by a hydrostatic pressure technique. Report on 43 cases. *Br J. Urol.* 1972;44(4):434-50.

[74] Garderet L, Bittencourt H, Sebe P, Kaliski A, Claisse JP, Esperou H, et al., Cystectomy for severe hemorrhagic cystitis in allogeneic stem cell transplant recipients. *Transplantation* 2000;70(12):1807-11.

[75] Droller MJ, Saral R, Santos G. Prevention of cyclophosphamide-induced hemorrhagic cystitis. *Urology* 1982;20(3):256-8.

In: Hematuria
Editors: Nikhil Vasdev and G. Boustead

ISBN: 978-1-63463-073-3
© 2015 Nova Science Publishers, Inc.

Chapter 3

Radiological Investigations of Haematuria

Michael McNeill, FRCR, Sebastian Mafeld, MBBS, and Philip Haslam, MRCP, FRCR, EBIR

Department of Radiology; Freeman Hospital,
High Heaton, Tyne & Wear, UK

Introduction

The role of imaging is central to the management of all patients requiring urological investigation of haematuria. Recent advances in technology have changed the way in which this is done in many centres worldwide, with CT coming to the forefront, though the fundamental challenge to seek the cause remains the same.

The causes of haematuria are myriad, ranging from benign and malignant to infectious and inflammatory conditions. This poses a diagnostic challenge, as it is often difficult to clinically assess which is most likely in any given scenario, and imaging strategies need to be able to evaluate a wide range of pathologies in a robust manner. These most commonly include calculi, renal masses, upper tract and bladder tumours, though there are many other abnormalities the radiologist needs to be aware of.

The following is a brief overview of main imaging techniques available.

Imaging Techniques

Plain Radiograph

The role of the plain KUB (kidneys; ureters; bladder) is somewhat limited, and it is really only in the detection of urinary tract calcification/calculi that it is of use. Its overall sensitivity for stone disease is in the range of 45-60%, therefore unenhanced CT has now become the gold standard for stone detection. [1 – 3]

Ultrasound

Ultrasound is a useful, often first-line investigation. It provides the most cost-effective method of imaging the urinary tract [4] with the added advantage of being radiation free, and therefore preferable for assessing young patients, pregnant women, and those who require regular follow up imaging. It is readily able to detect large renal masses, hydronephrosis, bladder tumours and large calculi. In experienced hands, small renal masses and urothelial tumours may also be identified, though it is widely recognised that the detection of small renal stones is less than 50%. Assessment of the ureters is usually not possible in most patients.

Intravenous Urogram

Historically the intravenous urogram (IVU), or excretory urography, has been the cornerstone of imaging the upper urinary tract. [1] Typically performed with a control film (for stone detection) intravenous contrast is injected, and subsequent serial plain films performed as contrast is excreted, to assess for focal filling defects in the pelvi-calyceal system, ureters and bladder. Tomography may also be performed, which uses sectional imaging through the body using a moving x-ray source, to provide an outline of the kidneys. The technique requires great skill in both the performing and reporting of the examination, with subtle abnormalities and secondary signs of pathology difficult to detect.

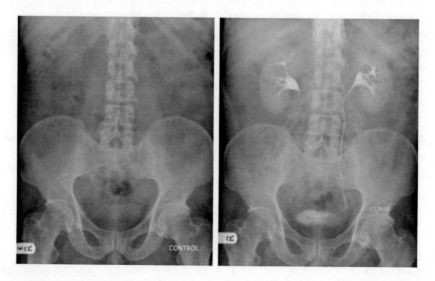

Figure 1. Control film and 15 minute film from a normal IVU series. This technique is becoming obsolete.

One of the main problems of intravenous urography with nephrotomography is the 67% sensitivity in detecting renal masses <3cm, even in the most experience hands, which is lessened still without tomography. [5] Images may be obscured by overlying bowel gas, and with more effective imaging techniques available, the use of IVU for the primary investigation into haematuria is waning.

Computed Tomography

Multi-detector CT urography (MDCTU) offers several advantages for imaging patients with haematuria: a multi-phase examination, with single breath-hold coverage of the abdomen, rapid acquisition and the ability for 2D and 3D reconstructions, to provide an in-depth and accurate depiction of the urinary tract and its associated pathologies.

Technique

Unenhanced images are initially obtained, to include the kidneys, ureters and bladder. Although the spatial resolution is less than that of plain film, it has far superior contrast resolution and is the optimal study to identify calcification. It is performed as a non-contrast study so that the high density of contrast media does not obscure small calculi as it is being excreted by the kidneys. This technique, even performed as a low dose study, will identify nearly all stones, with the rare exception of pure matrix calculi.

Following this, a bolus of intravenous contrast is administered, and images of the kidneys are acquired following a delay of approximately 100 seconds; i.e., a 'nephrographic phase'. This is the point at which each kidney is receiving as much contrast as it is excreting, thereby giving uniform enhancement of the cortex and medulla, optimising depiction of even small renal masses. During this phase, full imaging of the upper abdomen may be included in order to obtain post contrast detail of the remainder of the solid organs (particularly useful in the detection of metastatic disease when necessary).

In order to image the pelvi-calyceal system, ureters and bladder, a third delayed phase is performed, often with the use of an intravenous diuretic to increase urinary excretion of contrast, to therefore maximise the opportunity to detect filling defects. After a delay of approximately 8 – 10 minutes, images from the kidneys down to the bladder are again obtained, providing a detailed cross section of the upper tracts.

Some centres adopt a split bolus protocol in an attempt to reduce radiation dose. In this approach, a standard unenhanced CT is performed, and the subsequent nephrographic and delayed phase is carried out as a single acquisition using a 'split-bolus' of contrast – i.e., imaging at 100 seconds post contrast following a dose of IV contrast 8 – 10 minutes previously.

Typical Pathology

Urolithiasis

Unenhanced CT is highly accurate and sensitive in diagnosing stone disease as well as associated complications such as obstruction secondary to ureteric calculi. Difficulty may arise when imaging a very thin patient, where the ureters become difficult to trace low in the pelvis. However the delayed study will help to provide a road map as the ureters opacify, and this is seldom a problem in a three phase examination. Accurate information about the size, location and number of stones is easily obtained.

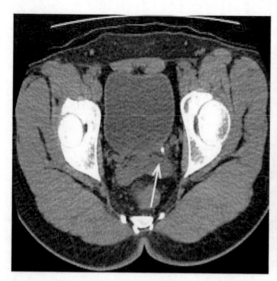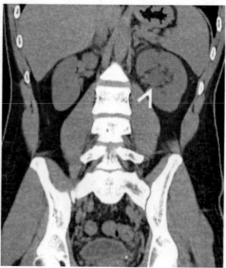

Figure 2. Small obstructing left vesico-ureteric calculus (arrow). Even on a single coronal image the moderate left hydronephrosis (arrow head) can be appreciated.

Neoplasms

Solid renal tumours will be best detected in the nephrographic phase, diagnosed when significant lesional enhancement is demonstrated. A mass is said to have enhanced significantly when its attenuation value has increased from the baseline pre-contrast study, by a value of more than 20 Hounsfield units (HU) – the density value used in CT. A lesion in question that demonstrates enhancement of less than 10HU is not considered significant, and between 10 – 20 HU indeterminate.

Upper tract tumours, commonly TCC, will be identified on the delayed phase as a filling defect in a contrast filled system, though the tumour itself may also demonstrate post contrast enhancement. With this in mind it is important to interrogate any such lesions on the initial two phases, as filling defects can also be due to benign causes such as thrombus.

Bladder tumours may be identified on the pre contrast and delayed phase scan, appearing as either a dense lesion or filling defect respectively. Small tumours may be difficult to appreciate, but this is seldom a problem as most patients will be having cystoscopic evaluation of the bladder.

Renal Cysts

Both the unenhanced study and nephrographic phase CT are useful to assess renal cysts. A simple renal cyst will be of fluid density, and demonstrate no significant post contrast enhancement. Bosniak describes a well known CT classification of more complex cysts, the detail of which is beyond the scope of this chapter. This relies on accurate assessment of fluid density, internal septations, areas of calcification, and the presence of enhancing components, the combination of which will determine malignant potential. All of these characteristics can be assessed accurately on the CT IVU.

Other Findings

Given that haematuria is often a non-specific sign or symptom, CT may also identify a number of other potentially related causes of blood arising from the urinary tract. There may be features of infection, particularly if complicated by pyelonephritis leading to abscess. Abnormal patterns of renal calcification may be suggestive of chronic infection such as TB. AV malformations, renal vein thrombosis and trauma are among other many causes of haematuria that can be identified on CT.

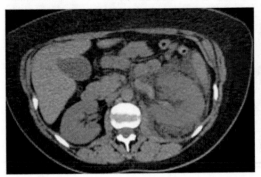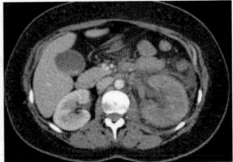

Figure 3. Left renal vein thrombosis on initial unenhanced CT, performed for renal calculi. Confirmed on subsequent post-contrast CT. (note the oedema around the left kidney and decreased enhancement).

Of course, there are potentially findings that will be entirely unrelated to the patient's symptoms. Given that post contrast images cover the liver and biliary system, pancreas, adrenals, GI tract, lung bases and skeleton, the possibility for extra-urinary findings is rather large. Often these incidental abnormalities are benign in nature, and can be discounted, though there may be a need for further investigation or follow-up.

A study by Weichung et al. found that up to 75% of patients imaged had extra-urinary findings. However, only 18% were shown to be clinically significant, with a small proportion having further imaging without a significant increase of overall per-patient costs. [6]

Imaging Strategy

Despite the many advantages of up to date technology and improved techniques, it is clear that not everyone with haematuria can be imaged with CT, and so a safe and reliable imaging strategy needs to be employed.

Haematuria is commonly subdivided into macroscopic and microscopic. The risk of malignancy in microscopic haematuria is much lower than with macroscopic haematuria, overall in the region of 9% in comparison to up to 30% respectively. [1] Many studies have evaluated patients presenting with haematuria, and studied the various population statistics with regard to final outcome. Edwards et al. found no cases of upper tract tumours below the age of 50 in men, and below 70 in women [7], whilst Khadra et al. concluded that no upper tract tumours were found in any patients under 40. There were, however, reported cases of bladder cancer in patients under 40. [8]

Based on studies such as these, the approach for imaging the patient with haematuria is similar in many centres. Our local protocol would advise cystoscopy in all cases of haematuria. In patients of any age with microscopic haematuria, additional investigation with ultrasound and x-ray KUB is suggested, proceeding to CT only if there are recurrent unexplained episodes, or if felt clinically high risk by the urologist.

Patients under 40 with macroscopic haematuria also undergo cystoscopy, ultrasound and x-ray KUB, with an additional CT KUB if there is associated loin pain. Further imaging with post contrast CT may be necessary if there are recurrent unexplained episodes.

Any patient over 40 with unexplained macroscopic haematuria has a higher risk of significant pathology and should have cystoscopy with three phase CT IVU.

Alternative Imaging Methods

MRI

Although CT is becoming the workhorse for the haematuria clinic, there are other methods to investigate the renal tract without the use of radiation. The role of MRI is ever increasing, and can be used in cases of compromised renal function, severe contrast allergy, young children and pregnant women. Furthermore it can be used as a problem-solving tool when CT is non-diagnostic. [9] The disadvantages include the higher cost involved, the time to acquire images, and the small bore nature of the scanner, meaning patients may find it claustrophobic.

Technique

Similar to CT, detail of the urinary tract can be obtained in multiple planes, thereby providing excellent overall detail. Standard protocols to assess renal lesions would usually include axial T1 and T2 imaging, with additional fat suppression and post contrast sequences. Imaging such as this will allow for the assessment of fat and water content within a lesion, and also accurately demonstrate any areas of enhancement. The latter tends to be more subjective than in CT, as an MR signal is not calibrated as density is in CT, but nevertheless, this has been shown to be accurate in detecting renal cell tumours. [10]

Uses

In cases where a small renal lesion demonstrates indeterminate enhancement on CT, MRI can be used at an interval to both follow up the lesion to assess for growth, as well as provide a second assessment of enhancement. This is also the case for complex renal cysts, which may have subtle internal features better depicted on MRI. In patients with suspected renal cell cancer, MRI may be useful to assess the presence of tumour thrombus in the renal vein or IVC, previously identified on CT. In cases where there will be an effect on the surgical approach, unlike bland thrombus, tumour thrombus will demonstrate enhancement, and so its true extent can be evaluated. Other uses of MRI include patients who are at increased risk for developing RCC, such as those with von Hippel-Lindau disease. These patients require regular, often annual follow up for the assessment of new enhancing renal tumours, and multiple CT scans would soon provide an unacceptable radiation burden, particularly in young patients. Excretory MR urography (MRU) will provide detail of the upper tracts and bladder in a similar manner to CT [11,12] and so is not commonly used. Diffusion weighted MRI is rapidly becoming standard practice in the assessment of prostate cancer, for which it is very helpful in finding focal tumours in locations commonly overlooked by biopsy, but such application in the kidney is of limited value, and again not commonplace in the assessment of renal lesions.

Contrast Enhanced Ultrasound

Standard grey-scale ultrasound is one of the most frequently used imaging methods, as is it safe, has no side effects and is widely available. The majority of asymptomatically diagnosed renal tumours are detected by ultrasound. Contrast enhanced ultrasound (CEUS) has gained clinical importance over recent years for its role in characterisation of hepatic lesions, where it has been shown to be highly accurate in the diagnosis of commonly encountered liver lesions. [13] Its use outside of the liver is less well documented, although 2011 EFSUMB (European Federation of Societies for Ultrasound in Medicine and Biology) guidelines gives great recognition to the potential of CEUS in the differentiation of solid and cystic renal lesions and characterisation of complex renal cysts. [14]

Technique

An intravenous injection of microbubbles is administered, each bubble approximately the size of a red blood cell. These circulate through the blood stream rapidly, and will cause tissue enhancement that is readily detectable by ultrasound, with the further advantage of being able to image the patient in real time. Other advantages include very low risk of allergy, low cost, no upper dose limit, and the fact that it has no adverse effect on nephron function, and therefore can be used in patients with even severe renal failure.

Uses

As in the liver, even the most subtle vascular supply to a lesion will be detected, and so the presence of an enhancing solid renal lesion will be easy to demonstrate. However, many of these lesions will be characterised with CT, due to the fact that even if a tumour is found incidentally on ultrasound, the patient will proceed to CT for full staging, at which point enhancement characteristics will be obtained.

However, its use in the assessment of complex renal cysts is probably the area of greatest potential. The Bosniak CT classification of a lesion is highly influenced by the presence or absence of enhancing tissue. Of the studies that have been performed, it is recognised that CEUS may 'over call' the presence of enhancing components due to its high sensitivity to vascularity, which may lead to the upgrading of a lesion. The true accuracy of this is yet to be fully studied, and remains a potential for large scale multicentre trial. If proven to be reliable CEUS would very well suited to the follow up of indeterminate lesions and could potentially replace CT in this regard. [14]

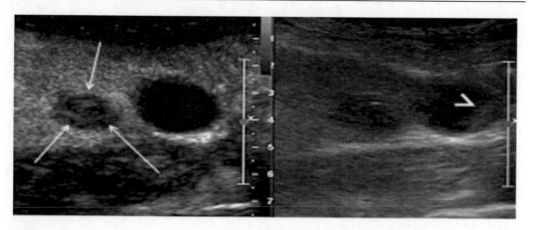

Figure 4. Non-enhancing haermorrhagic renal cyst adjacent to an enhancing cystic neoplasm in a patient with VHL. The left hand image is the contrast enhanced scan, and shows enhancement in the septations in the lesion on the left. The right side cyst has haemorrhage in it which doesn't enhance.

References

[1] Van der Molen AJ, Hovius MC. Haematuria: A Problem-Based Imaging Algortihm Illustrating the Recent Dutch Guidelines on Haematuria. *AJR*; 198:1256-1265.

[2] Levine JA, Neitlich J et al. Urethral calculi in patients with flank pain: correlation of plain radiography with unenhanced helical CT. *Radiology* 1997; 204:27-31.

[3] Ege G, Akman H et al. Can computed tomography scout radiograph replace plain film in the evaluation of patients with acute urinary tract colic? *Acta Radiol* 2004; 45:469-473.

[4] Israel GM, Casalino DD, et al. Indeterminate renal masses. *ACR Appropriateness Criteria.* 2010.

[5] Amendola MA, Bree RL et al. Small renal cell carcinomas: resolving a diagnostic dilemma. *Radiology.* 1988; 166(3):637-641.

[6] Liu W, Mortele KJ et al. Incidental extraurinary findings at MDCT urography in patients with haematuria: prevalence and impact on imaging costs. *AJR* 2005; 185: 1051-1056.

[7] Edwards TJ, Dickinson AJ et al. A prospective analysis of the diagnostic yield resulting from the attendance of 4020 patients at a protocol-driven haematuria clinic. *BJU Int* 2006; 97;301-305.

[8] Khadra MH, Pickard R et al. A prospective analysis of 1930 patients with haematuria to evaluate current diagnostic practice. *J Urol* 2000; 163:524-527.

[9] Nikken JJ, Krestin GP. MRI of the kidney - state of the art. *Eur Radiol* 2007; 17:2780-2793.

[10] Middleton W, Dodds W, et al. Renal calculi: sensitivity for detection with ultrasound. *Radiology* 1988; 167:239-244.

[11] Regan F, Kuszyk B, et al. Acute ureteric calculus obstruction: unenhanced spiral CT versus HASTE MR urography and abdominal radiograph. *Br J Radiol* 2005: 78;506-511

[12] ˙Sudah M, Vanninen R et al. MR urography in evaluation of acute flank pain: T2-weighted sequences and gadolinium-enhanced three-dimensional FLASH compared with urography. Fast low-angle shot. *AJR Am J Roentgen.* 2001; 176:105–112

[13] Ignee A, Straub B et al. Contrast enhanced ultrasound of renal masses. *World J Radiol* 2010: 28; 2(1):15-31.

[14] Piscaglia F, Nolsoe C et al. The EFSUMB Guidelines and Recommendations on the Clinical Practice of Contrast Enhanced Ultrasound (CEUS): Update 2011 on non-hepatic applications. *Ultraschall in Med* 2012; 33:33-59.

In: Hematuria
Editors: Nikhil Vasdev and G. Boustead

ISBN: 978-1-63463-073-3
© 2015 Nova Science Publishers, Inc.

Chapter 4

Role of Interventional Radiology in Haematuria

Frances Colgan, FRCR, Sebastian Mafeld, MBBS,
and Philip Haslam, MRCP, FRCR, EBIR
Department of Radiology; Freeman Hospital,
High Heaton, Tyne & Wear, UK

Introduction

Interventional Radiology offers a wide variety of treatment options in patients with haematuria and urological malignancy. Active bleeding can be embolised safely and effectively from a percutaneous approach, obviating the need for more invasive surgery. Renal cell tumours can be ablated percutaneously in patients who are not suitable for nephron-sparing surgery. Bone metastases from renal cell tumours can be ablated from a percutaneous approach, or embolised prior to surgical resection in order to reduce the intra-operative blood loss. Whilst this chapter concentrates on the management of haematuria it is important to remember that interventional radiology is not confined to endovascular approaches and that patients with renal and ureteric obstruction often attend the IR department for other procedures, such as nephrostomy and ureteric stent placement.

Embolisation in Haematuria

Embolisation is the generic term given to the mechanical blocking of a blood vessel. In the context of haematuria this can be used selectively in the management of active arterial bleeding and for the symptomatic control of haematuria in the intermediate and longer term. Access to the arterial system is normally gained via a percutaneous common femoral artery puncture and the vessel supplying the tumour is cannulated under fluoroscopic guidance using a guidewire and catheter. Embolic agents are deployed into the target under x-ray screening.

Embolic agents come in a variety of forms including liquids (cyanoacrylate glue; onyx; gelfoam made into slurry); particles (bland or drug-coated); coils and plugs. The choice of embolic agent is influenced by the size of, and the flow in, the vessel to be embolised.

Embolisation is usually performed by an interventional radiologist. These procedures are performed under screening guidance so additional environmental factors must also be considered, such as the availability of high quality fluoroscopic equipment, a radiographer and skilled nurses.

Endovascular intervention is the treatment of choice for most cases of active bleeding, offering fast, effective and minimally invasive treatment with a significant reduction in the mortality and morbidity associated with open surgery. The interventional radiologist should be involved at an early stage to facilitate the logistics of transferring the patient to a suitable environment. Often these patients will undergo CT scanning in order to confirm the diagnosis and the location of haemorrhage and plan the likely treatment. When active bleeding is confirmed, the images should be discussed with the interventional radiologist.

Angiomyolipoma

Angiomyolipoma (AML) is a histologically benign mixed connective tissue tumour containing vascular, muscle and fatty elements. It most commonly occurs sporadically and in isolation, but in a small number of patients it is associated with the neurocutaneous syndromes of Tuberous Sclerosis and neurofibromatosis. Whilst small lesions are often asymptomatic, larger lesions carry an increased risk of spontaneous haemorrhage. These patients may present with sudden onset of acute flank pain and haemodynamic shock in keeping with retroperitoneal bleeding. In this situation, providing the patient is stabilised, embolisation provides an effective, nephron-sparing approach to haemostasis compared with open surgery. Sometimes patients present with intermittent pain due to multiple small bleeds and these patients can also be treated with embolisation.

Emergency Embolisation

As AMLs are often asymptomatic, many patients will present with flank pain and shock of an unknown cause and the diagnosis will be made on CT (figure 1.). When active bleeding is confirmed the case should be discussed with an interventional radiologist with a view to percutaneous embolisation. The patient should be transported to the fluoroscopy suite (or theatres with screening capability) with anaesthetic team support to deal with any current or future haemodynamic compromise. The embolisation itself is a minimally invasive procedure normally performed under local anaesthetic or, in some cases, conscious sedation. The patient should be consented for damage to the access vessels (including pseudoaneurysm formation); renal loss; and sequelae resulting from non-target embolisation (i.e., mis-placement of embolic material).

Percutaneous access is gained to the common femoral artery using either manual palpation or ultrasound guidance and a guidewire is placed in the descending aorta. The catheter and guidewire are then manipulated into the main renal artery on the side of the AML and digitally subtracted fluoroscopic images are obtained to delineate the renal arterial anatomy and identify the source of bleeding. Superselective catheterisation is then performed and the embolic agent is deployed as close as possible to the target to stop the bleeding whilst minimising the loss of normal renal tissue (figure 2). One common pitfall is arterial spasm, which can make the bleeding point more difficult to find, but which can be managed with the administration of intra-arterial nitrate. If a patient has multiple renal arteries, selective catheterisation of each in turn may be required if the bleeding point has not been identified at the first attempt and also because the AML may be supplied by more than one vessel. If no bleeding point is demonstrated, further recourse to the CT scan should be undertaken, to confirm the anatomy and to exclude an alternative site of bleeding. In some situations the bleeding points cannot be identified and selective segmental embolisation of the kidney may be performed.

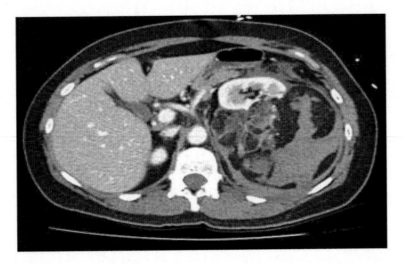

Figure 1. CT demonstrating a ruptured AML. Note the fatty component to the tumour and the associated haematoma.

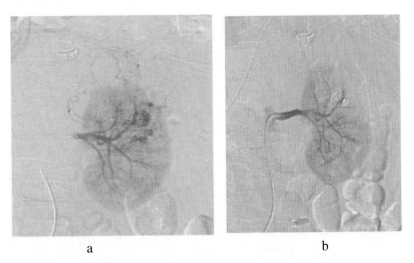

a   b

Figure 2. (a) subtracted angiographic runs demonstrating arterial supply to tumour and (b) subsequent embolisation.

Prophylactic Treatment Options

For patients in whom the AML is known about prior to any haemorrhage, decisions can be made to embolise these electively, to reduce risk of subsequent bleeding. Ideally this would be undertaken at the point at which the risk of morbidity associated with likelihood of bleeding is greater than the risks associated with the procedure itself. The decision to electively embolise such patients should be made within the context of a multi-disciplinary team discussion with careful consideration of the likelihood of bleeding in relation to its size and the specific risks of treatment. In these patients super-selective embolisation should be performed to preserve as much functioning renal parenchyma as possible. Prophylactic embolisation is a similar endovascular procedure to that undertaken in ruptured AML. Patients with multiple AML and repeated episodes of bleeding may require repeated embolisation.

Longer Term Outcomes

Patients known to have a predisposition to AML should be seen by a specialist in that field, and in the case of familial neurocutaneous syndromes, referral to a clinical geneticist may be appropriate.

Renal Cell Carcinoma

Owing in part to advances in imaging techniques over the past 20 years, there has been a decrease in the mean tumour size of renal cell carcinoma (RCC) at the time of detection. During the same time interval, more traditional surgical approaches have been replaced with minimally invasive techniques including partial nephrectomy, and laparoscopic and robot-assisted techniques. These techniques make use of advances in haemostatic techniques (ligaclips, floseal and surgical bolster) and bring with them a spectrum of new post-operative imaging findings and complications for the interventional and diagnostic radiologists. Percutaneous tumour ablation is a minimally invasive technique performed under imaging guidance by interventional radiologists and has a comparable outcome to conventional operative intervention in the management of small renal tumours.

Complications of Renal Surgery

Common complications of both renal surgery and imaging guided percutaneous biopsy include haemorrhage and urine leak, both of which can often be managed in the IR department. Haemorrhage can be due to inadequate intra-operative haemostasis, pseudoaneurysm formation and/or inadvertent (and sometimes initially unrecognised) damage to adjacent structures, for example the splenic artery, with retractors or laparoscopic instruments. A similar set of complications occur with image-guided biopsy.

Patients who are bleeding post-operatively should undergo early cross-sectional imaging to identify the likely source of bleeding and thus allow targeted catheterisation under screening guidance. After the decision has been made to proceed to the IR department, close attention should be paid to the patient's haemodynamic status, as aggressive fluid resuscitation, early transfusion and anaesthetic support may be necessary. The culprit vessel should be identified on catheter angiogram, guided by the CT findings and embolised with appropriate material (figure 3). After haemostasis, nearby vessels should also be checked to ensure there is not a second source of haemorrhage. If the patient remains unstable then further cross sectional imaging and diagnostic catheter angiography, with or without further embolisation may be required.

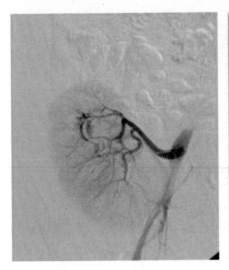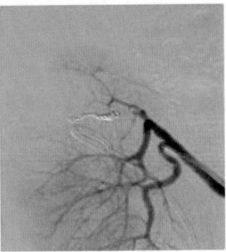

Figure 3. (a) active bleeding from a branch renal artery in a transplant kidney after a renal biopsy. (b) selective embolisation has been performed via the right external iliac artery.

Pre-Operative Arterial Embolisation of RCC

Pathological fracture through metastatic RCC is often fixed surgically, with adjuvant pre-operative embolisation to aid haemostasis. Embolisation is performed as described above and normally 24 hours prior to the orthopaedic surgery.

Ablation for RCC

Percutaneous tumour ablation can be performed by the interventional radiologist as a form of nephron-sparing intervention. A probe is located into the centre of the tumour from a percutaneous approach under imaging guidance (figure 4.). Energy is then applied to the tumour to cause cell death. This energy can be radiofrequency or microwave energy, cryotherapy and more recently irreversible electroporation (IRE). These techniques are most successful in small tumours (less than 4cm) and those which are distinct from nearby structures, in order to minimise the risk of collateral damage. Use of 'hydrodissection', the displacement of adjacent structures from the target area by the instillation of fluid or gas in order to limit injury is commonly practised. At the time of imaging-localisation of the tumour for ablation, a biopsy can also be taken, the result of which will guide future follow-up.

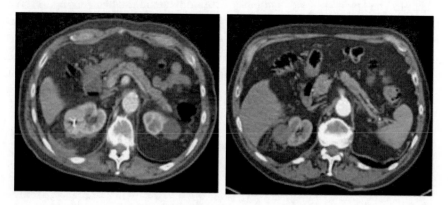

Figure 4. (a) small right RCC containing radiofrequency probe during ablation (b) one month post-ablation images showing some residual tumour but with no remaining enhancement indicating successful ablation.

Bladder Haemorrhage

Intractable bladder haemorrhage has a variety of causes in the oncological and post-operative situations including TCC, prostatic carcinoma, cystitis (haemorrhagic, radiotherapy and chemotherapy-induced and chronic urinary tract infection). The clinical presentation is normally related to the haematuria. Patients may present with frank haematuria or pain associated with clot retention, persisting anaemia with or without a transfusion requirement or in the case of a large volume acute haemorrhage, with hypovolaemic shock. These patients are often poor surgical candidates and endovascular management, where it is possible, carries a smaller risk than that of conventional surgery. The morbidity associated with persistent haematuria includes quality of life issues, prolonged hospital episodes and the risks associated with repeated blood transfusion.

Management of Bladder Haemorrhage

After any haemodynamic instability has been corrected, the patient presenting with haematuria should normally undergo an assessment of coagulation function; bladder washout (with large bore irrigation catheters); pharmacological attempt at haemostasis where appropriate (tranexamic acid) and in some situations an attempt may be made at direct haemostasis with alum/silver nitrate or formalin bladder irrigation.

After this initial management it may be appropriate to proceed to transurethral tumour resection (TURT); radiotherapy or embolisation to achieve longer-term haematuria control. Radiotherapy can be performed in the outpatient setting if the patient is stable but can take a few days to become effective. It is worth bearing in mind that patients having non-definite treatment for haematuria will often experience further episodes of bleeding.

Bladder Embolisation

Bladder embolisation, like embolisation for other sites remains a minimally invasive procedure, it is relatively low risk and suitable for most patients. The source of bleeding is usually the anterior division of the internal iliac artery, and the principles remain the same i.e., to embolise as selectively as possible in order to limit the likelihood of the complications. Super-selective embolisation is preferred when a bleeding point is identified. When no culprit vessel is demonstrated, tumour neo-vascularisation (tumour blush) should guide embolisation, and the embolic agent instilled into the appropriate branch vessel under screening guidance. In cases where no definite bleeding point or tumour is demonstrated, bilateral anterior divisions of the internal iliac arteries may be embolised. This approach carries with it a higher incidence of complication and associated morbidity including buttock claudication and necrosis if the inferior gluteal arteries are embolised. In the endovascular management of bladder haemorrhage, the principles remain the same – embolise just enough to control bleeding whilst limiting local damage. A combination of coils and particulate embolic agents are often used.

Future Perpectives: Loin Pain – Haematuria Syndrome

Loin pain haematuria syndrome is a relatively rare condition comprising intermittent loin pain with episodic visible or non-visible haematuria. It is more common in female patients and its aetiology is poorly understood. Several methods have been used to try and control the pain from this syndrome including nerve block techniques, surgical denervation, capsulotomy and autotransplantation, but as yet there is no generally accepted effective treatment.

Renal artery denervation is an endovascular treatment whereby the sympathetic nerve supply to the kidney, which runs along the renal artery, is destroyed using catheter-based ablation. The use of this technique has been tried in the management of loin-pain-haematuria syndrome but at the time of writing no formal evaluation of this use has been undertaken.

References

Abt D, Bywater M, Engeler DS, Schmid H-P. Therapeutic options for intractable hematuria in advanced bladder cancer. *International Journal of Urology* (2013) 20, 651–660

Baumann C, Westphalen K, Fuchs H, Oesterwitz H, Hierholzer J. Interventional Management of Renal Bleeding after Partial Nephrectomy. *Cardiovasc Intervent Radiol* (2007) 30:828–832

Becker F, Siemer S, Humke U, Hack M, Ziegler M, Stockle M. Elective nephron sparing surgery should become standard treatment for small unilateral renal cell carcinoma: Long-term survival data of 216 patients. *Eur Urol* (2006) 49(2):308–313 de Beus E, Blankestijn PJ, Fox JG, Zoccali C. Catheter-based renal denervation as a novel treatment for loin pain haematuria syndrome. *Nephrol Dial Transplant* (2013) 28: 2197–2199

Breen DJ, Rutherford EE, Stedman B, Roy-Choudhury SH, Cast JEI, Hayes MC, Smart CJ. Management of Renal Tumors by Image-Guided Radiofrequency Ablation: Experience in 105 Tumors. *Cardiovasc Intervent Radiol* (2007) 30:936–942

Chang YH, Wang LJ, Chuang CK et al. The efficacy and outcomes of urgent superselective transcatheter arterial embolization of patients with ruptured renal angiomyolipomas. *J Trauma* (2007) 62:1487–1490

Esler MD, Krum H, Schlaich M et al. Renal sympathetic denervation for treatment of drug-resistant hypertension: one-year results from the symplicity HTN-2 randomized, controlled trial. *Circulation* 2012; 126: 2976–2982

Ginat DT, Saad W, Davies M, Walman D, Erturk E. Bowel displacement for CT-guided tumor radiofrequency ablation: techniques and anatomic considerations. *J Endourol* 2009; 23(8):1259–1264

Halpenny D, Snow A, McNeill G, Torreggiani WC. The radiological diagnosis and treatment of renal angiomyolipoma - current status. *Clinical Radiology* 65 (2010) 99–108

Incedayi M, Turba UC, Arslan B, Sabri SS, Saad WEA, Matsumoto AH, Angle JF. Endovascular Therapy for Patients with Renal Angiomyolipoma Presenting with Retroperitoneal Haemorrhage. *Eur J Vasc Endovasc Surg* (2010) 39, 739-744

Kaufmann JA, Lee MJ. Vascular and Interventional Radiology: The Requisites (Expert Consult - Online and Print), 2e (Requisites in Radiology). *Elsevier* 2013, 978-0323045841.

Kessel D, Ray C. Transcatheter Embolization and Therapy (Techniques in Interventional Radiology). *Springer* 2009, 978-1848008960.

Lee SY et al. Embolization of Renal Angiomyolipomas: Short-Term and Long-Term Outcomes, Complications, and Tumor Shrinkage. *Cardiovasc Intervent Radiol* (2009) 32:1171–1178

Liguori et al. Intractable haematuria: long-term results after selective embolization of the internal iliac arteries. *BJU International* (2010) 500-503.

In: Hematuria

Editors: Nikhil Vasdev and G. Boustead

ISBN: 978-1-63463-073-3

© 2015 Nova Science Publishers, Inc.

Chapter 5

Hematuria in Autosomal Dominant Polycystic Kidney Disease: Etiology, Management and Long-Term Prognosis

Alma Idrizi[1,]*, Myftar Barbullushi[1], Alketa Koroshi[1],
Nereida Spahia[1] and Enton Kaçulini[1]

[1]Department of Internal Medicine, Service of Nephrology,
University Hospital Center "Mother Teresa", Tirana, Albania

Introduction

Autosomal dominant polycystic kidney disease (ADPKD) is a multisystemic and progressive disorder characterized by the formation and enlargement of cysts in the kidney and other organs (e.g., liver, pancreas, spleen). Clinical features usually begin in the third to fourth decade of life, but cysts may be detectable in childhood and in utero [1].

Hematuria is one of the most important renal manifestations in ADPKD [2] with two distinguished forms of clinical presentation: microhematuria and gross hematuria. Patients are considering having microhematuria if the urinalysis showed up to 5 red blood cells per high power field seen with a microscope and gross hematuria if they gave a history of observing blood in the urine.

Gross hematuria is the presenting symptom in 15–20 per cent and occurs at least once in 30–50 per cent of patients with ADPKD (Table 1) [3, 4].

Hematuria usually occurs prior to loss of kidney function, and may be the presenting symptom of the disease [4, 5]. A precipitating event, such as a urinary tract infection or strenuous activity, can often be identified prior hematuria and recurrent episodes are not uncommon [4]. It occurs less frequently in PKD2 than in PKD1 patients [6]. Its incidence increases with the degree of kidney enlargement. Gross hematuria is usually secondary to

---

* Tel.: +355684063625/Fax: +35542363644, E-mail: alma_idrizi@yahoo.com.

renal cyst rupture into the renal pelvis. It may follow strenuous physical activity or minor trauma but often occurs spontaneously.

Table 1. Clinical manifestations of ADPKD

Manifestations	Prevalence (%)
Renal	
Hypertension	60 before renal failure
	90 at ESRD
Pain (acute and chronic)	60
Gross hematuria	50
Urinary tract infection	Men 20; women 70
Calculus	20
Renal failure	≅50 by age 70
Hepatobiliary	
Asymptomatic liver cysts	80 at age 60
Symptomatic polycystic liver disease	Uncommon (male : female ratio 1 : 10)
Congenital hepatic fibrosis	Rare
Caroli disease	Rare
Cardiovascular	
Mitral valve prolapse	25
Intracranial aneurysm	8
Intracranial dolichoectasia	2
Ascending aortic dissection	Rare
Other	
Pancreatic cyst	9
Arachnoid cyst	8
Hernia	Rare
Inguinal	13
Umbilical	7

ADPKD - autosomal dominant polycystic kidney disease, ESRD - end stage renal disease.

Propensity to cyst bleeding is explained by the rich vascular network of cyst walls, including aneurysmal vessels and neoformation of capillaries [7]. The fact if it is micro or gross hematuria depends to the existence or non-existence of a communication between the bleeding cyst and the collecting system. Bleeding into a cyst that does not communicate with the urinary system may not produce visible blood; in this setting, patients typically have localized flank pain and, in some cases, a low grade fever. Depending on the amount of bleeding, intracystic haemorrhage can produce transient moderate fever and leucocytosis in the absence of infection [8]. Gross hematuria rarely lasts for more than 7 days [4].

Gross hematuria, together with other factors can cause the abdominal pain. Acute pain is suggestive of intracystic haemorrhage, urinary tract obstruction (by clot or stone), or infection (associated with fever) (Table 2) [8].

Table 2. Specific causes of acute abdominal pain in patients with ADPKD

Cause	Frequency	Fever
Renal		
Cyst bleeding	+++	Mild (<38°C, max 2 days) or none
Stone	++	With pyonephrosis (rare)
Infection	+	High, prolonged with cyst involved
Liver		
Cyst infection	Rare	High, prolonged
Cyst bleeding	Very rare	Mild (<38°C, max 2 days) or none

ADPKD - autosomal dominant polycystic kidney disease.

Chronic pain, often described as abdominal discomfort and fullness, is frequently observed.

Infection, segmental renal infarction, and passage of renal calculi also cause gross hematuria in ADPKD patients [8].

Late-onset and/or prolonged or recurrent hematuria should also raise the possibility of an unrelated problem such as bladder cancer, especially in patients with increased risk factors for this neoplasm. Prolonged or recurrent hematuria, particularly in a man over the age of 50, raises the possibility of an underlying renal cell carcinoma [5] or of an unrelated problem such as bladder cancer or IgA nephropathy [9].

Etiology of Gross Hematuria in ADPKD

The main cause of gross hematuria in ADPKD is intracystic haemorrhage (with or without pain). Rupture of a cyst into the collecting system is thought to be responsible for the development of hematuria. Renal cysts in ADPKD are associated with excessive angiogenesis evinced by fragile vessels stretched across their distended walls [8]. When traumatized, these vessels may leak blood into the cyst, causing it to expand rapidly, resulting in excruciating pain. If bleeding continues, then the cyst may rupture into the collecting system, causing gross hematuria. Alternatively, the cyst may rupture into the subcapsular compartment and eventually dissect through the renal capsule to fill the retroperitoneal space. Although hemorrhage into a cyst is also common, the typical presentation is pain rather than hematuria since many cysts do not communicate with the collecting system [5]. The hematuria due to cyst rupture generally resolves within two to seven days with conservative therapy consisting of bed rest and hydration, analgesics that excluding nonsteroidals, and in some cases holding antihypertensive medications [4]. Occasionally, bleeding can persist for several weeks. With unusual and severe bleeding, percutaneous arterial embolization or even nephrectomy may become necessary [10].

In a study performed in 180 patients, Idrizi et al. [11] found gross hematuria present in 113 patients (63%): 67 patients were females (16 of them underwent to renal loss), and 46 were males (12 of them underwent to renal loss). In 39 patients gross hematuria was due to renal cyst rupture into the renal pelvis. In 43 patients gross hematuria was diagnosed before age 30 (38%), while in 70 patients it was diagnosed after age 30 (62%).

In many times gross hematuria is associated with urinary tract infection [11].

Nephrolithiasis is another cause of hematuria, usually microscopic, in patients with ADPKD. The hematuria should resolve with passage or removal of the stone. In these cases, the flank or abdominal pain is presenting symptom in 30 per cent of the patients and occurs at some time in at least 50–60%, its frequency increasing with age and with the size of the cysts [3].

In a study of Idrizi et al. [12], 65 patients (56%) with kidneys stones reported episodes of gross hematuria. In 40% of patients the presence of stones was associated with a history of urinary tract infections and flank pain.

There is a potential risk of cyst rupture and traumatic hemorrhage because of shockwave lithotripsy for urinary calculi in ADPKD, although it is reported to be a safe and effective treatment option. Sometimes the nephrectomy is performed [13].

In some cases the gross hematuria can occurs in ADPKD patients with sickle–cell disease. Metabolic or environmental changes such as hypoxia, acidosis, dehydration, hyperosmolality or hyperthermia may transform silent sickle–cell trait into a syndrome resembling sickle–cell disease with vaso–occlusive crisis due to an accumulation of low deformable red blood cells in the microcirculation originating hematuria from papilar necrosis. On the other hand, it has been demonstrated an earlier onset of end–stage renal disease (ESRD), in blacks with ADPKD and sickle–cell trait when compared with blacks with ADPKD without the trait. Co–herence of sickle–cell trait may have influence on ADPKD evolution to ESRD and other complications, such as cystic haemorrhages [14].

In contrast to macroscopic hematuria, microscopic hematuria (especially with red blood cells casts) is rarely seen in ADPKD patients. Therefore, the detection of proteinuria in the nephrotic range, hematuria with red blood cells casts, and/or a rapid decline of renal function in ADPKD patients suggest the possibility of superimposed glomerular diseases [15].

If hematuria is recurrent or persists for more than two weeks should also raise the possibility of an unrelated problem with cysts such as bladder cancer, especially in patients with increased risk factors for this neoplasm [16]. Renal malignancies do not occur in a greater frequency in ADPKD patients than they do in the general population [17]. In our study, four patients with gross hematuria were associated with renal malignancy in computed tomography (CT) scanning [12].

Fispathology of Gross Hematuria in ADPKD

Mild trauma can lead to intrarenal hemorrhage or bleeding into the retroperitoneal space accompanied by intense pain that often requires narcotics for relief [18]. Spontaneous cyst bleeding is important to consider in this particular group of patients; it can be prolonged by local activation of fibrinolysis by urokinase [19]. The cysts are associated with excessive angiogenesis evinced by fragile vessels stretched across their distended walls. When traumatized, these vessels may leak blood into the cyst, causing it to expand rapidly, and provoking frightening pain. If bleeding continues, then the cyst may rupture into the collecting system, causing gross hematuria. Alternatively, it may rupture into the subcapsular compartment and eventually dissect through the renal capsule to fill the retroperitoneal space. In massive bleeding, the blood may reach the skin that covers the flank and abdomen, where it is recognized as subcutaneous ecchymoses (Gray-Turner sign) [18].

How We Can Detect the Gross Hematuria?

Acute cyst hemorrhage and infection can be identified from symptoms, laboratory data, and CT/ magnetic resonance imaging (MRI) findings. Distinguishing between infection and cyst hemorrhage is often challenging, and the diagnosis relies mainly on clinical and bacteriologic findings. Increased white blood cells more than 10.000/µl, serum C-reactive protein >15.0mg/dl, and temperature degree more than 38°C suggest cyst infection [20]. All of the cysts with hemorrhage contained a high-density mass-like area or showed overall high density on CT, and all patients with cyst hemorrhage had abdominal pain or gross hematuria.

The intracystic haemorrhages in the kidney may be diagnosed by using ultrasound, CT scanning or MRI. However, diagnosis is difficult in the presence of a persistent, but very slight haemorrhage.

Ultrasound

Ultrasound is an excellent choice for repeated imaging as it is fast, relatively inexpensive and lacks ionising radiation. It is able both to suggest the diagnosis and to assess for cyst complications.

Cysts with haemorrhage or infection will demonstrate echogenic material within the cyst, without internal blood flow. Calcification may develop. Renal cell carcinomas in contrast, although usually cystic in the setting of ADPKD, will have solid components of thick septae with blood flow) [21].

CT Scanning

CT scanning appears to be superior to ultrasonographic images in helping to assess retroperitoneal rupture of a cyst and perinephric extension of blood or pus from an infected cyst. [22, 23].

On the other hand, positron emission tomography-CT allows us to distinguish haemorrhages from cystic infection [24-26]. Evidence from CT scanning suggests that intracystic haemorrhage, shown as hyperdense subcapsular cysts, is present in 90% of patients with ADPKD [5, 27].

There are often dozens of superficial cysts that may cause intracystic haemorrhage. Direct inspection of the "hyperdense" subcapsular cysts, from CT scanning, has revealed cysts to be filled with cellular debris derived from the breakdown of blood products [27].

Hemorrhagic cysts are often considered radiologically indeterminate. The increase in CT attenuation of renal cysts complicated by hemorrhage has been attributed to clot retraction, with resultant concentration of protein components of blood [28, 29], and to an elevated iron content [30]. Other reports suggest that alterations of attenuation values may occur with highly proteinaceous cyst contents [31] and with transient iodine accumulation [32, 33].

MRI

The imaging technique of MRI may observe intracystic haemorrhages that would never have been noticed before. This is an important step forward, since it is widely known that patients with ADPKD who suffer from frequent hematuria episodes or show signs of intracystic haemorrhage develop chronic renal failure more quickly [34, 35].

MRI is especially useful for examining patients who are allergic to iodinated contrast media and those with compromised renal function who are at risk for iodinated contrast–induced renal failure.

MRI has demonstrated homogeneous high signal intensity in hemorrhagic cysts on both T1 - and T2-weighted spin-echo images [36]. The T1 and T2 reported were variable, but always less than those for simple cysts.

Multiple factors are likely to contribute to the overall signal intensity in hemorrhagic cyst. Such factors may include serum hematocrit and protein levels, stage of clot retraction, concentration of oxidized iron (Fe^{+3}) in hemoglobin, and composition of cyst fluid (e.g., osmolarity, water content, protein content, and cholesterol content). Correlations among MRI, MR spectroscopy, and chemical analysis may provide insight into the characterization of cyst fluid as well as other body fluids [37].

Management of Hematuria

Treatment options for controlling severe haemorrhage from polycystic kidneys are limited [14, 38, 39]. The episodes of hematuria are normally managed with conservative medical treatment with bed rest, hydration, analgesics, blood transfusion, correction of coagulopathies, embolisation, erythropoietin stimulating protein and rarely require surgery. Nonetheless, other modalities have been tried to avoid prolonged hospitalization and nephrectomy and to preserve kidney function. These include other antifibrinolytic agents such as aprotinin and epsilon aminocaproic acid (EACA) [19] and more recently, tranexamic acid (trans-4-(aminomethyl) cyclohexanecarboxylic acid) [40, 41]. It is a synthetic lysine analogue with strong anti-fibrinolytic activity. The plasminogen binds to fibrin to form plasmin, which in turn breaks down fibrin molecules into fibrin degradation products. Tranexamic acid blocks plasminogen's lysine binding sites and prevents its interaction with fibrin. As a fibrinolysis inhibitor, it is 7 to 10 times more potent than epsilon aminocaproic acid. Some clinical trials have proven it to reduce blood loss in patients with primary menorrhagia and those who have undergone cardiopulmonary bypass surgery, prostatectomy, hip replacement and liver transplant procedures [42]. It was recently reported to be effective in treating hematuria in patients with sickle-cell anemia as well [43]. Tranexamic acid is well-tolerated in general. Although a few cases of renal cortical necrosis have been reported, [44, 45] its side effects are mainly gastrointestinal and include nausea, vomiting, diarrhea and abdominal pain. Myoclonus and encephalopathy due to overdose have been described in only one case [46]. Tranexamic acid is excreted through glomerular filtration, and therefore accumulates in the presence of low renal function. Patients with CRF will require dose titration. On the other hand, the effectiveness of hemodialysis in tranexamic acid elimination has not been studied [47, 48].

The normal dose is 10mg/kg given 3 or 4 times daily. Andersson et al. [49] recommend reducing dosages in patients with decreased renal function as follows: for serum creatinine levels of 120-250μmol/l (1.36-2.83mg/dl), 10mg/kg IV twice daily; for serum creatinine levels of 250-500μmol/l (2.83-5.66mg/dl), 10mg/kg IV once daily; for serum creatinine levels ≥500μmol/l (5.66 mg/dl), 10mg/kg IV every 48 hours. Similar doses have been used with good results in patients on dialysis with upper digestive tract haemorrhage [48]. Treatment options for controlling severe hemorrhage from polycystic kidneys are limited [14, 38, 39, 50, 51]. As far as we are aware, there have been only two published studies of tranexamic acid as treatment for hematuria due to cyst bleeding in ADPKD, and both were isolated cases [40, 41]. In one of the cases, the initial dose was 20mg/kg IV, which was later maintained by the oral route [40]. Peces et al. suggest that in the most severe cases of uncontrolled hemorrhage it would be reasonable to administer anti-fibrinolytic treatment with tranexamic acid [52]. The patients received doses ranging from 15mg/kg 3 times daily IV to 10mg/kg 3 times daily orally with treatment lasting between 2 and 5 days. All courses of treatment were equally effective. No side effects were observed at any time. However, they recommend administering oral or IV tranexamic acid at the lowest possible effective dosage and during the shortest possible period in order to lessen the risk of adverse effects. It is possible that treatment lasting less than 3 days could be just as effective, but this type of dose was not studied. Lastly, early at-home use of tranexamic acid by patients with ADPKD and recurrent hematuria could be very cost-effective if it prevented the need for hospitalisation. The main limitations of the study of Peces et al. are a small sample size and the lack of an untreated control group [52]. So, tranexamic acid may be used safely in selected ADPKD patients with severe or intractable hematuria that does not respond to conventional treatment. The drug can be administered orally or intravenously, and the dose must be adjusted in patients with kidney failure. Treatment with tranexamic acid in ADPKD may preserve renal function both directly, by stopping cyst bleeding and decreasing the frequency of hematuria episodes, and indirectly, by preventing embolisation and/or nephrectomy [52].

For patients with large kidneys with many cysts, decortication (deroofing and collapse of cysts) surgery has been performed, either open or more recently laparascopic [53] with similar results with respect to the number of cysts unroofed (150–200) and the proportion of patients with pain relief (60–70 per cent at 2 years), but also with a similar quite high rate of complications (37–47 per cent) including haemorrhage and urine leakage.

Very rarely, bleeding may be severe and persistent, notably in dialyzed patients, necessitating uninephrectomy [1].

Long-Term Prognosis of Hematuria in ADPKD

Renal hemorrhage caused by cysts occurs at any age and diminishes the quality of life. Although they are self-limiting, successive episodes of gross hematuria may have a detrimental effect on renal function in the long term [54, 35]. Gross hematuria is associated with more rapid progression of kidney disease in ADPKD [4]. Gross hematuria is more likely among individuals with larger kidneys (particularly when >15 cm in length), hypertension and higher plasma creatinine concentrations [4, 55]. Frequent episodes of gross hematuria before the age of 30 may be associated with worse renal outcomes; this may possibly reflect accelerated cyst expansion [54]. Patients with a history of renal hemorrhage evinced by repeated episodes of gross hematuria have the largest kidneys (Table 3) [4, 54] and progress to renal insufficiency faster than those without this history.

In a retrospective clinical study, Gabow et al. [4] found that male athletes who had ADPKD and participated in contact sports had more hematuric episodes and developed renal insufficiency sooner than those who did not participate.

In the study of Idrizi et al. [11] having at least one episode of gross hematuria before age 30 was associated with a worse renal survival than not having such an episode (10-year difference in renal survival; $P < 0.001$) (Figure 1). The difference in survival for those who had gross hematuria before age 30, compared with those who did not have this experience, was significant either for women (Figure 2) or men (Figure 3) (the difference in 10 years renal survival, $p < 0.001$ and 12-year, $p < 0.001$ respectively). These data suggest that patients with recurrent episodes of gross hematuria may be at risk for more severe renal disease since the mean age of the first episode of hematuria occurred on average at 30 years, considerably earlier than renal functional deterioration occurs.

Table 3. Relation between kidney volume and variables

Variables	Number Studied	Volume Method	Mean Kidney Volume			
			With variable	Without variable	P Value	Reference
Proteinuria	270	US	1190 ± 93	578 ± 32	<0.0001	[8]
Microalbuminuria	49	US	853 ± 87	535 ± 52	<0.01	[8]
Hypertension		US				[5]
Males	76		624 ± 47	390 ± 43	<0.0005	
Females	89		446 ± 32	338 ± 24	<0.002	
Hypertension	43	CT	976 ± 472	739 ± 311	<0.05	[84]
	241	MR	628 ± 48	352 ± 33	<0.0001	[80]
Hypertension children	62	US	2.7 ± 2.3	1.2 ± 2.5	<0.05	[85]
Hypertension children	70	US	125 ± 7	83 ± 6	<0.0001	[42, 43]
Gross hematuria	**191**	**US**	**820 ± 87**	**588 ± 52**	**<0.03**	**[3]**
Progressive loss of renal function	43	CT	895	606		[84]
	220	US	598 ± 368	366 ± 168	<0.0001	[77]

US- ultrasound, CT- computed tomography MR- magnetic resonance.

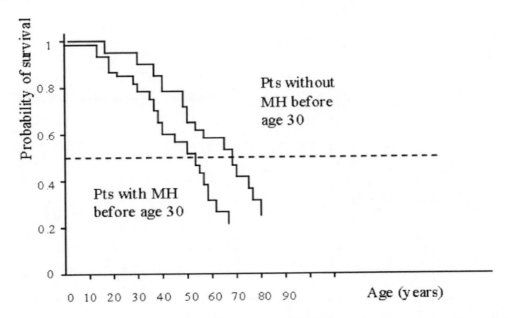

Figure 1. Renal survival in patients with macrohematuria (MH) before age 30 vs. patients without MH before age 30.

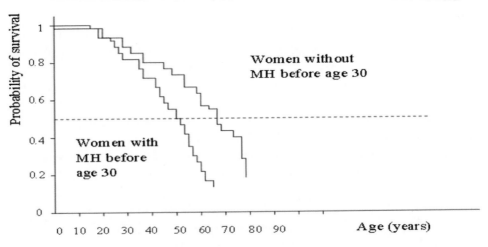

Figure 2. Renal survival in women with macrohematuria (MH) before age 30 vs. women without MH before age 30.

Hematuria after Renal Transplant

Hematuria must be investigated fully and promptly in the ADPKD population, as one would for the general population, to exclude a renal tract malignancy. Native nephrectomy is not routinely indicated in ADPKD patients undergoing transplantation but is reserved mainly for those with recurrent infection and pain. Hematuria in such patients should not be assumed to be of benign origin and requires exclusion of urinary tract malignancy as the incidence of renal cell carcinoma in this population is at least as common as in the general population [56].

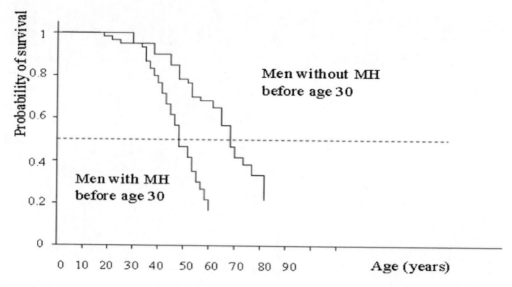

Figure 3. Renal survival in men with macrohematuria (MH) before age 30 vs. men without MH before age 30.

Conclusion

Hematuria is one of the most important renal manifestations in ADPKD, being the presenting symptom in 15–20% of patients. Gross hematuria is a common manifestation of PCKD. It can result from trauma, renal calculi, tumor, or infection. The intracystic haemorrhages in the kidney may be diagnosed by using ultrasound, CT scanning or MRI. The episodes of hematuria are normally managed with conservative medical treatment with bed rest, hydration, analgesics, blood transfusion, correction of coagulopathies, embolisation, erythropoietin stimulating protein, antifibrinolytic agents. Very rarely, bleeding may be severe and persistent, notably in dialyzed patients, necessitating uninephrectomy. Gross hematuria is associated with more rapid progression of kidney disease in ADPKD.

References

[1]   Wilson P. D. Polycystic kidney disease. *N. Engl. J. Med.*, Jan. 8 2004; 350 (2): 151-64.
[2]   Kaehny W. D., Gabow P. A. Polycystic kidney disease: Clinical, radiologic and genetic approaches to problems in diagnosis, in Narins RG (ed): Contemporary Issues in Nephrology: Diagnostic Techniques in Renal Disease. New York, NY, Churchill Livingstone 1992; 47-72.
[3]   Milutinovic J., Fialkow P. J., Agodoa L. Y. et al. Autosomal dominant polycystic kidney disease: Symptoms and clinical findings. *Q. J. Med.*, 1984; 212: 511-522.
[4]   Gabow P. A., Duley I., Johnson A. M. Clinical profiles of gross hematuria in autosomal dominant polycystic kidney disease. *Am. J. Kidney Dis.*, 1992; 20: 140-143.
[5]   Gabow P. A. Autosomal dominant polycystic kidney disease. *N. Engl. J. Med.*, 1993;329(5):332.

[6]   Bello-Reuss E., Holubec K., Rajaraman S. et al. Angiogenesis in autosomal dominant polycystic kidney disease. *Kidney Int.,* 2001;60:37–45. [PubMed]

[7]   Hateboer N., Bogdanova N., Dijk M. et al. Comparison of Phenotypes of Polycystic Kidney Disease Types 1 and 2. European PKD1-PKD2 Study Group. *Lancet,* 1999;353: 103–7.

[8]   Oxford Textbook of Clinical Nephrology by Martin Barratt, Alex M. A. Davison, J. Stewart Cameron and Jean-Pierre Grunfeld (6 Jan. 2005).

[9]   Dedi R., Bhandari S., Turney J. H. et al. Lesson of the week: Causes of hematuria in adult polycystic kidney disease. *BMJ,* 2001;323(7309):386-387.

[10]   Ubara Y., Katori H., Tagami T. et al. Transcatheter renal arterial embolization therapy on a patient with polycystic kidney disease on hemodialysis. *Am. J. Kidney Dis.,* 1999;34(5):926.

[11]   Idrizi A., Barbullushi M., Petrela E. et al. The influence of renal manifestations to the progression of autosomal dominant polycystic kidney disease. *Hippokratia,* 2009;13(3):161-164.

[12]   Idrizi A., Barbullushi M., Gjata M. et al. Prevalence of nephrolithiasis in polycystic kidney disease, *Central European Journal of Medicine,* 2011; 6 (4): 497-501.

[13]   Kim H. G., Bae S. R., Lho Y. S. et al. Acute cyst rupture, hemorrhage and septic shock after a shockwave lithotripsy in a patient with autosomal dominant polycystic kidney disease. *Urolithiasis,* 2013;41(3):267-269.

[14]   Peces R., Peces C., Cuesta–López E. et al. Co-herencia de poliquistosis renal autosómica dominante y hemoglobina con rasgo falciforme en afroamericanos. *Nefrología,* 2011; 31(2):162-168.

[15]   Sumida K., Ubara Y., Hoshino J. et al. Myeloperoxidase-antineutrophil cytoplasmic antibody-associated crescentic glomerulonephritis in autosomal dominant polycystic kidney disease. *BMC Nephrology,* 2013; 14:94.

[16]   Bennett W. M., Elzinga L. W. Clinical management of autosomal dominant polycystic kidney disease. *Kidney Int.,* 1993; 44: Suppl. 42: S74-S79.

[17]   Anderson G. A., Degroot D., Lawson K. Polycystic Renal Disease. *Urology,* 1993; 2 (4): 358-364.

[18]   Levine E., Grantham J. J.: Perinephric hemorrhage in autosomal dominant polycystic kidney disease: CT and MR findings. *J. Comput. Assist. Tomogr.,* 1987;11:108-111.

[19]   Zwettler U., Zeier M., Andrassy K. et al. Treatment of gross hematuria in autosomal dominant polycystic kidney disease with aprotinin and desmopressin acetate. *Nephron,* 1992;60(3):374.

[20]   Suwabe T., Ubara Y., Sumida K., Clinical features of cyst infection and hemorrhage in ADPKD: new diagnostic criteria. *Clin. Exp. Nephrol.,* 2012 Dec.;16(6):892-902.

[21]   Nahm A. M., Henriquez D. E., Ritz E. Renal cystic disease (ADPKD and ARPKD). *Nephrol. Dial. Transplant.,* 2002;17 (2): 311-314.

[22]   Antiga L., Piccinelli M., Fasolini G. et al. Computed tomography evaluation of autosomal dominant polycystic kidney disease progression: a progress report. *Clin. J. Am. Soc. Nephrol.,* Jul. 2006;1(4):754-760.

[23]   Perrone R. Imaging progression in polycystic kidney disease. *N. Engl. J. Med.,* May 18 2006;354(20):2181-2183.

[24] Chen J. H., Wu S. T., Wu C. C. Autosomal dominant polycystic kidney disease with cystic haemorrhage and infection. *Acta. Clin. Belg.*, 2010;65:446-447.

[25] Piccoli G. B., Arena V., Consiglio V. et al. Positron emission tomography in the diagnostic pathway for intracystic infection in ADPKD and "cystic" kidneys. A case series. *BMC Nephrol.*, 2011;12:48.

[26] Jouret F., Lhommel R., Beguin C. et al. Positron-emission computed tomography in cyst infection diagnosis in patients with autosomal dominant polycystic kidney disease. *Clin. J. Am. Soc. Nephrol.*, 2011;6:1644-1650.

[27] Levine E., Grantham J. J. High-density renal cysts in autosomal dominant polycystic kidney disease demonstrated by CT. *Radiology*, 1985;154:477-482.

[28] Sussman S., Cochran S. T., Pagani J. J., et al. Hyperdense renal masses: a CT manifestation of hemorrhagic renal cysts. *Radiology*, 1984;1 50:207-211.

[29] New P. F. J., Aronow S. Attenuation measurements of whole blood and blood fractions in computed tomography. *Radiology*, 1976;121 :635-640.

[30] Curry N. S., Brook G., Metcalf J. S. et al. Hyperdense renal mass: unusual CT appearance of a benign renal cyst. *Urol. Radiol.*, 1982;4:33-35.

[31] Fishman M. C., Pollack H. M., Arger P. H. et al. High protein content: another case of CT hyperdense benign renal cyst. *J. Comput. Assist. Tomogr.*, 1983;7: 1103-1106.

[32] Mayer D. P., Baron A. L., Pollack H. M. Increase in CT attenuation values of parapelvic renal cysts after retrograde pyelography. *AJR*, 1982;139:991-993.

[33] Shanser J. D., Hedgcock N. W., Korobkin M. Transit of contrast material into renal cysts following urography or arteriography. *AJR*, 1978;130:584.

[34] Masoumi A., Reed-Gitomer B., Kelleher C. et al. Developments in the management of autosomal dominant polycystic kidney disease. *Ther. Clin. Risk Manag.*, 2008;4: 393-407.

[35] Grantham J. J., Torres V. E., Chapman A. B., CRISP Investigators. Volume progression in polycystic kidney disease. *N. Engl. J. Med.*, 2006;354:2122-2130.

[36] Le-Strake L., VanDerHem G. A., Hooijkaas J. A. P. Nuclear magnetic resonance imaging of the kidney. *Diagn. Imag. Clin. Med.*, 1984;53: 198-202.

[37] Hilpert P. L., Friedman A. C., Radecki P. D. MRI of Hemorrhagic Renal Cysts in Polycystic Kidney Disease. *AJR*, 1986;146: 1167-1172.

[38] Reay E. K., McEleny K., McDonald S. et al. Blunt renal trauma in adult polycystic kidney disease and the use of nephron sparing selective arterial embolization. *J. Trauma*, 2009;66:564-566.

[39] Bae K. T., Grantham J. J. Imaging for the prognosis of autosomal dominant polycystic kidney disease. *Nat. Rev. Nephrol.*, 2010;6:96-106.

[40] Vujkovac B., Sabovic M. A successful treatment of life-threatening bleeding from polycystic kidneys with antifibrinolytic agent tranexamic acid. *Blood Coagul. Fibrinolysis*, 2006;17:589-591.

[41] Alameel T., West M. Tranexamic acid treatment of life-threatening hematuria in polycystic kidney disease. *Int. J. Nephrol.*, 2011;2011:203579.

[42] Rannikko A., Petas A., Taari K. Tranexamic acid in control of primary hemorrhage during transurethral prostatectomy. *Urology*, 2004;64:955-958.

[43] Davis N. F., McGuire B. B., Lawlor L. et al. Oral tranexamic acid as a novel treatment option for persistent haematuria in patients with sickle cell disease. *Ann. Hematol.*, 2010;89:1179-1180.

[44] Koo J. R., Lee Y. K., Kim Y. S. et al. Acute renal cortical necrosis caused by an antifibrinolytic drug (tranexamic acid). *Nephrol. Dial. Transplant.*, 1999;14:750-752.

[45] Odabaş A. R., Cetinkaya R., Selçuk Y. et al. Tranexamic-acid-induced acute renal cortical necrosis in a patient with haemophilia A. *Nephrol. Dial. Transplant.*, 2001;16:189-190.

[46] Hui A. C., Wong T. Y., Chow K. M. et al. Multifocal myoclonus secondary to tranexamic acid. *J. Neurol. Neurosurg. Psychiatry*, 2003;74:547.

[47] Sabovic M., Zupan I. P., Salobir B. et al. The effect of long-term, low-dose tranexamic acid treatment on platelet dysfunction and haemoglobin levels in haemodialysis patients. *Thromb Haemost.*, 2005;94:1245-1250.

[48] Sabovic M., Lavre J., Vujkovac B. Tranexamic acid is beneficial as adjunctive therapy in treating major upper gastrointestinal bleeding in dialysis patients. *Nephrol. Dial. Transplant.*, 2003;18:1388-1391.

[49] Andersson L., Eriksson O., Hedlund P. O. et al. Special considerations with regard to the dosage of tranexamic acid in patients with chronic renal diseases. *Urol. Research,* 1978;6:83-88.

[50] Peces R., Peces C., Pérez-Dueñas V. et al. Rapamycin reduces kidney volume and delays the loss of renal function in a patient with autosomal-dominant polycystic kidney disease. *Nephrol. Dial. Transplant. Plus,* 2009;2:133-135.

[51] Peces R., Peces C., Cuesta-López E. et al. Low-dose rapamycin reduces kidney volume angiomyolipomas and prevents the loss of renal function in a patient with tuberous sclerosis complex. *Nephrol. Dial. Transplant.*, 2010;25:3787-3791.

[52] Peces R., Aguilar A., Vega C. et al. Medical therapy with tranexamic acid in autosomal dominant polycystic kidney disease patients with severe haematuria. *Nefrologia,* 2012;32(2):160-165.

[53] Dunn M. D., Portis A. J., Naughton C., et al. Laparoscopic marsupialization in patients with autosomal dominant polycystic kidney disease. *J. Urol.,* 2001;165:1888-1892.

[54] Johnson A. M., Gabow P. A. Identification of patients with autosomal dominant polycystic kidney disease at highest risk for end-stage renal disease. *J. Am. Soc. Nephrol.*, 1997;8(10):1560-1567.

[55] Milutinovic J., Fialkow P. J., Agodoa L. Y. et al. Clinical manifestations of autosomal dominant polycystic kidney disease in patients older than 50 years. *Am. J. Kidney Dis.,* 1990;15(3):237-243.

[56] Patel P., Horsfield C., Compton F. et al. Native nephrectomy in transplant patients with autosomal dominant polycystic kidney disease. *Ann. R. Coll. Surg. Engl.*, 2011 July; 93(5): 391-395.

In: Hematuria
Editors: Nikhil Vasdev and G. Boustead

ISBN: 978-1-63463-073-3
© 2015 Nova Science Publishers, Inc.

Chapter 6

Glomerular Causes of Hematuria: Causes and Workup

Samir Gautam and Emaad M. Abdel-Rahman[*]

Division of Nephrology, University of Virginia,
Charlottesville, Virginia, US

Introduction

Blood in the urine is hematuria, when it is macroscopic it can be frightening to the patients and when it is microscopic can be challenging to the practitioner. Glomerular hematuria usually presents as microscopic hematuria, although it can present as macroscopic hematuria too. [1]

Microscopic hematuria is defined as presence of 3 red blood cells (RBCs) or more per high power field in a spun of urine sediment [2,3]. Macroscopic hematuria, on the other hand, is defined as a hematuria when there is more than 1 cc of blood in the urine, or visible change in the color of urine. [3]

The key to diagnosing glomerular hematuria is the presence of dysmorphic red blood cells and red blood cell casts. Presence of proteinuria with hematuria favors a glomerular source for the hematuria. The epidemiology of glomerular hematuria may be difficult to ascertain as it can be challenging to differentiate from other non-glomerular hematuria and usually requires an expert to collect and review the urinary sediment. [4] The most common causes for non-glomerular hematuria are upper urinary tract causes (as nephrolithiasis, pyelonephritis, polycystic kidney disease) or lower urinary tract causes (as cystitis, prostatitis, urethritis and cancer of bladder or prostate).

---

[*] Corresponding author: Emaad M Abdel-Rahman, MD, PhD, FASN, Professor of Nephrology, Address: Box 800133, Nephrology Division, UVA, Charlottesville, VA 22908, Phone: (434) 243-2671, Fax (434) 924-5848, Email: ea6n@virginia.edu

Pathogenesis

The glomerular hematuria is caused by the breach of glomerular basement membrane. In cases of nephritis it is caused by severe inflammation of the glomerular capillaries thereby causing osmotic, mechanical and enzymatic damage to the RBCs giving rise to its dysmorphic shape. [5, 6] As the RBC comes out through the basement membrane, there is distortion in the integrity of the cells. [5, 6] At times, these cells attach to the matrix protein and give a microscopic appearance of a cast. [5, 6]

Etiology and Clinical Presentation

Grossly, glomerular hematuria can be divided into isolated hematuria or nephritic syndrome (Figure 1). [4] Isolated hematuria occurs without any other urine abnormalities (absence of infection, proteinuria) [4], while nephritic causes of hematuria can be part of a syndrome that include hypertension, worsening renal function, non-nephrotic range proteinuria, edema and oliguria. While IgA nephropathy and thin basement membrane disease are the most common causes of isolated hematuria [4], nephritic hematuria can be caused by a wide range of pathologies (Figure 1).

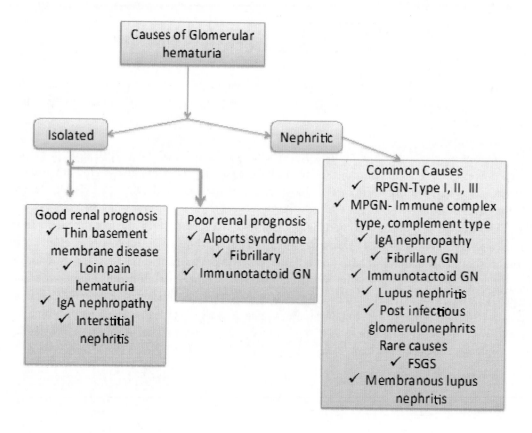

Figure 1.

I. Isolated asymptomatic Hematuria

1. IgA Nephropathy

IgA nephropathy is the most important glomerular cause of macroscopic hematuria. [1] It is also the most common glomerular disease worldwide. [7, 8]

Patients with IgA nephropathy can present with various variety of hematuria from macroscopic to microscopic, isolated to nephritic, acute kidney injury as well as chronic kidney injury. IgA nephropathy is usually associated with upper respiratory tract infection, where it may be cyclical with each bout of respiratory tract infection. It also may be associated with Henoch-Schonlein purpura (HSP). [7, 9] Although IgA nephropathy is a disease of children, recently it has been seen in elderly people with staphylococcus infection where mesangial IgA deposits are seen by immuno- fluorescence examination of renal tissue. The outcome of this variant is variable, but sometimes it improves after the treatment of staphylococcus infection. [10]

Increasingly IgA nephropathy is recognized as an autoimmune entity. The presence of poorly galactosylated IgA1 in the serum is postulated to be the trigger for the formation of IgA autoantibodies and formation of immune complexes and deposition in the mesangium. [8, 11]

Examining a renal biopsy wherein the light microscopy may show mesangial expansion and by immunofluorescence there can be IgA deposits alone or along with other immuno-globulins could show this. [11]

Prognosis of IgA nephropathy is variable where 20-40 % of patients with this disease may develop end stage renal failure after a prolonged course of up to 20 years. Several risk factors may be able to predict mortality or the need for dialysis, and these include proteinuria more than 1 gm/24 hours urine, hypertension and severe histological findings. [12, 13] Crescent formation is rare. Approximately 50-60% of histological recurrence of IgA nephropathy occurs after 5 years of transplantation.

Blood pressure control, reduction of proteinuria usually with angiotensin converting enzyme inhibitor (ACEi)/Angiotensin receptor blocker (ARB), and fish oil are the main core of treatment. However, in more severe cases, steroid and cyclophosphamide can be considered.

2. Thin Basement Membrane Disease

Thin basement membrane disease or benign familial hematuria is a common cause of asymptomatic microscopic hematuria. [1, 4]

The disease can rarely present with macroscopic hematuria along with flank pain and it mostly occurs during a bout of upper respiratory tract infection. The patients with thin basement disease may have mild proteinuria with no abnormalities in the renal function. [1, 4, 14]

Family history may be positive for the disease and it usually lasts a lifetime. [1, 4, 14].

Patients with thin basement disease have abnormal collagen type IV and along with Alports syndrome they are known as collagen IV nephropathies. [15]

The only medical indication for renal biopsy for suspected thin basement membrane disease is when the patient is being considered as a transplant donor. The patients have excellent renal prognosis. The diagnosis is made on the basis of electron microscope findings as the light microscope might be normal.

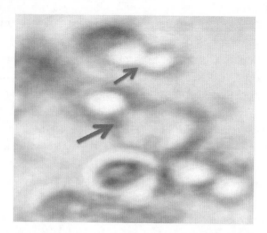

Figure 2. Published by: Samir Gautam/Rahman, Dysmorphic Red blood cells (Micky Mouse appearance). These cells are typically seen in glomerular hematuria.

3. Alport Syndrome (AS)

AS is also known as hereditary nephritis. Though patients with AS may have isolated hematuria, the disease may lead to end stage renal failure. [14] Early detection of the disease is necessary to manage the patients other extra-renal manifestations as blood pressure and the associated chronic kidney disease. [4, 15, 16]

Alport syndrome is a disease of the glomerular basement membrane (GBM) but instead of only showing thin GBM as in thin basement membrane disease, GBM is lamellated and at times thin also. [15-17]. Patients with Alport syndrome may have sensori-neural hearing loss, hematuria and renal failure, as well as a family history of renal failure. [15, 16] It is caused by a defect in the gene encoding for type IV collagen proteins, namely the genes encoding for alpha 3, 4, 5 subunits of collagen IV.

The common mode of inheritance is mostly X-linked, although autosomal dominant and autosomal recessive variants may also be found. Initial presentation may be microscopic hematuria but as the age progresses there is worsening hematuria, proteinuria, hypertension and renal failure.

II. Nephritic Syndrome

1. IgA Nephropathy: Discussed Above

2. Post infectious Glomerulonephritis

Post infectious GN (PIGN) is a relatively new phenomenon. Until three decades ago most of the post infectious glomerulonephritis were in the form of post streptococcal glomerulonephritis. [18-20] However, recently this type of glomerulonephritis is identified with other types of infection. Pharyngitis or skin infections with group A beta hemolytic streptococcus usually precedes the renal failure. Staphylococcal glomerulonephritis is more recognized, however, other microbial organisms can also lead to post infectious glomerulonephritis. [18-20]

On microscopic examination of a renal biopsy of a patient with PIGN, there is immune complex deposition in the sub-endothelial portion of the glomerulus. This is more prevalent in alcoholic, cirrhotic and/or immunosuppressed hosts. In addition to features of nephritis, these patients will also have low complement C3 and C4. Clinical suspicion of post streptococcal glomerulonephritis usually does not require a renal biopsy unless other causes of rapidly progressive glomerulonephritis (RPGN) are suspected. Steroids have limited role. Treating infection is the main stay of management of PIGN. [18, 19, 21]

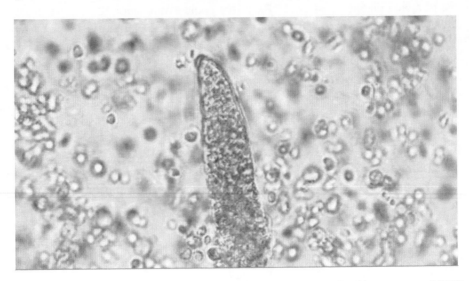

Figure 3. Published by: Samir Guatam/ Rahman. Active sediment, as defined by presence of RBC casts. Presence of RBCs within the matrix. The above sediment was seen in a middle aged ma with Lups Nephritis.

3. Membrano-Proliferative Glomerulonephritis (MPGN)

Membrano-proliferative glomerulonephritis or mesangio-capillary glomerulonephritis is a variant of glomerulonephritis which is classified by its histology. It is the third or fourth common cause of glomerulonephritis leading to end stage renal failure. The presentation is very heterogonous, starting for asymptomatic hematuria to nephritis to RPGN. It also may present with minimal proteinuria or nephrotic range proteinuria.

The histology of the disease may vary depending upon the clinical course. In the past the classification was based on electron microscope findings of immune complex deposits, primary (Idiopathic, type I- sub endothelial deposits, type II-deposits in the GBM and type III- subepithelial and subendothelial deposits), as well as and secondary depending on the associated conditions like hepatitis C. With recent understanding of the complement mediated pathway, MPGN is divided into 2 subtypes, immune complex mediated (type I) and complement mediated (Type II). [22, 23]

Hypocomplementemia is present in both types of MPGN, mostly there is low C3 and normal C4 in complement medicated. [22, 23]

Type I or Immune complex mediated MPGN is mainly a disease of the classical complement pathway. There is immune complex deposition and mesangial expansion. The antigenic trigger can be from a chronic infection (commonly hepatitis C, Cryoglobulinemia), or gammopathies. [24, 25]

Type 2 or complement mediated: It is mainly through activation of alternative complement cascade and most of the times there is low C3 and normal C4. [22, 23]

4. Rapidly Progressive GN (RPGN)

Rapidly progressive glomerulonephritis (RPGN), present with cola or brown colored urine and are associated with rapid deterioration of renal function. RPGN is defined as doubling of serum creatinine within 8- 12 weeks. It is a clinical diagnosis not a pathological diagnosis. It is only diagnosed after careful microscopic examination that shows dysmorphic RBCs (fig 2) and/or RBCs casts (fig 3), proteinuria and rapid deterioration of renal function. [13, 26] Renal biopsy of patients with RPGN shows crescent and the percentage of crescents are helpful as prognostic indicator. [19]

RPGN encapsulates wide variety of pathologies, and can be subdivided in various categories depending upon the type of disease processes. Three subtypes of RPGN has been described I, II and III.

a. Anti-GBM Disease (AGBM)

Good pastures syndrome or Anti-glomerular baseline membrane disease is also known as Type I RPGN, which may present with only renal failure or in combination with pulmonary symptoms. Anti-GBM antibodies are identified. [27-29]

These are the antibodies against type IV collagen. It is temporally related to chemical, infection or inhalation exposure. The disease, if not identified and treated early, may lead to end stage renal failure. [28-30]

b. Immune complex-mediated

Immune complex mediated glomerulonephritis or type II RPGN involves immune complex deposition diseases, with the main one being lupus nephritis. Lupus nephritis can be the first presenting feature of systemic lupus erythromatosus (SLE) or at times the SLE patients during the course of disease develops lupus nephritis and in the immunofluorescence it presents as 'full house". [31]

The diagnosis of lupus nephritis is based on clinical and laboratory analysis. Clinically, the patient will have systemic symptoms of SLE along with positive antinuclear antibodies, low complements mainly C4, hematuria and proteinuria. [31, 32]

The second important cause of type II RPGN is post infectious, mostly post streptococcal but it can occur with other viral and bacterial infections, as described above.

c. Pauci-Immune GN

Pauci immune glomerulonephritis or type III. The term 'Pauci-Immune' was coined as there is no immune complex deposition detected by immuno-fluorescence or electron microscopy. [27] The common disease process in this category is granulomatous polyangiitis previously known as Wegener's disease, Churg-Strauss syndrome and microscopic polyangiitis. [27] Pauci-immune GN can present as renal- pulmonary syndrome, but presence of both system diseases is not necessary for diagnosis. They may or may not be associated with antibodies but most of the times they are associated with anti-myeloperoxidase and anti-proteinase-3 antibodies as almost 5% of the cases have false positive tests .[33, 34] Antibodies are directed against the neutrophils and their interaction causes damage, which is seen as crescents in the renal biopsy. [27]

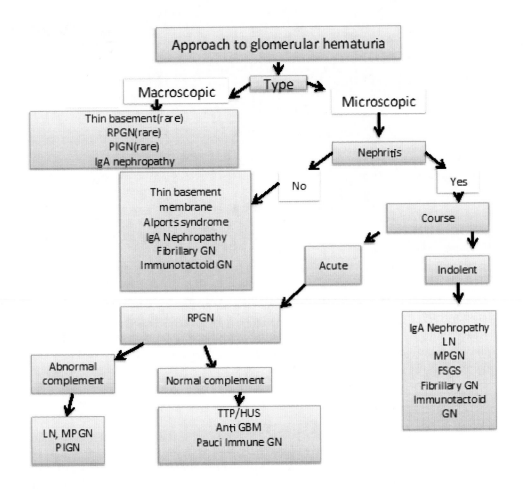

Figure 4.

5. SLE Nephritis

SLE nephritis or Lupus Nephritis could be classified into five different sub classification namely, minimal mesangial, mesangial proliferative, focal lupus nephritis, diffuse lupus nephritis and membranous lupus nephritis. [31, 33]

This classification is based on kidney biopsy findings. While type I is clinically undetectable, type II may have microscopic hematuria, and type III, type IV, and type V are severe forms presenting with hematuria, severe proteinuria and abnormal renal function. [31, 33] Lupus nephritis type IV can present as RPGN as described above. [31,33]

6. Focal Segmental Glomerular Sclerosis (FSGS)

FSGS is a rare cause of hematuria, and most of the times it is a secondary type of FSGS, which gives hematuria. Figure 4 is the algorithm for the diagnosis and table 1 shows the summary of glomerular hematuria.

Table 1. Distinct features of some types of Glomerular Hematuria

Disease	Complement	Serology
Thin basement membrane	Normal	Normal
Loin pain hematuria	Normal	Normal
Lupus Nephritis	Low C3, Low C4(preferentially suppressed)	ANA+, AntiSmith+, Anti DSDNA+
Good Pastures syndrome	Normal	Anti-GBM antibody
Fibrillary and Immunotactoid GN	Normal	Normal
Pauci-Immune GN	Normal	ANCA-MPO and PR-3
IgA Nephropathy	Normal	Increased serum IgA levels (sometimes)
Alports Syndrome	Normal	Normal
Post infectious Glomerulonephritis	Both Low	Anti DNAse B and ASO positive for post streptococcal
MPGN- Immune complex type	Both low (Classical complement cascade)	Positive for various infections esp. Hep C, Cryo, various autoimmune disorders, gammopathies
MPGN- complement mediated type	Only C3 low esp. in C3GN, normal C4	Normal

MPO: Myeloperoxidase, PR-3: Proteinase-3,

7. Fibrillary and Immunotactoid GN

Patients with fibrillary and immunotactoid glomerulonephritis may present with isolated hematuria, or nephritic or nephrotic syndrome and they are resistant to most of the treatment and progress to End stage renal disease. [35].

Diagnosis

Certain clues can be helpful in the diagnosis of glomerular hematuria, but at times the definite diagnosis can be difficult even after performing a renal biopsy. The color of urine is not usually bright red or pink in contrast to non-glomerular hematuria. [13] Glomerular hematuria is mostly associated with some degree of proteinuria, usually more than 300 mg but not within the nephrotic range. [4] The glomerular hematuria is uniform throughout the urine sample and it does not clot in contrast to the urological hematuria. [13]

There are certain disease processes or serological markers that may trigger glomerular hematuria , top in the list for example, hemoptysis, joint pain, rashes, renal failure, abnormal complements, hypoalbuminemia, history of lupus, leukemia, family history of renal dysfunction, recent history of any infections etc.

The diagnosis of glomerular hematuria requires a systematic approach, starting from thorough history taking, physical examination, urinalysis, to obtaining chemistries, serologies, and occasionally a renal biopsy. [4] In addition to the hematuria, the presence of proteinuria, a renal ultrasound to rule out urological causes of hematuria, and the presence of abnormal renal function are helpful in defining glomerular hematuria.

While isolated glomerular hematuria can be followed by routine monitoring of renal function and proteinuria by primary care physician every 6 months, [4] it is reasonable for the primary provider to seek urgent referral to nephrologist whenever microscopic hematuria is present with proteinuria and abnormal renal function. [4]

Presence of RBC cast is classical for glomerular hematuria but its absence doesn't exclude glomerular hematuria. [4, 36, 37] Identifying RBC casts can be challenging as, the examination of the cast should be from the fresh sediment as the matrix denatures. [5,6] If unable to find the RBC casts, then there should be dysmorphic RBCs. [4,36,37]

Urological bleeding can have less than 20% of dysmorphic RBCs. [2] Phase contrast microscopy also has a great utility in diagnosing glomerular hematuria. [17] It can detect acanthocytes in the urine sediment. [17].With dysmorphic RBCs of more than 35% the sensitivity is 69-100% whereas the acanthocytes of more than 5% have sensitivity to detect glomerular hematuria between 88-100%. [17]

While certain diseases as IgA and thin basement membrane disease may require renal biopsy to achieve definite diagnoses, the diagnosis of other diseases may be based on clinical judgment. Although RPGN is a clinical diagnosis, the nephrologist will need to distinguish between each subtype. In this aspect, in addition to obtaining a good history and physical examination and examining urinary specimen, serological analysis can be helpful (Table 1) Anti-GBM antibodies are present in Good Pasture syndrome while anti myeloperoxidase and proteinase antibodies can be present in pauci immune glomerulonephritis. [26, 30, 33, 34]

In Lupus Nephritis, the complements will be low while the anti-double stranded DNA (ADsDNA) activity will be high. [31, 32] Patients with post streptococcal glomerulonephritis will have low complements and a positive anti- streptococcal antibody. [18, 19, 37]

The patients with MPGN will have low complements, either both or one of them. [26] While the presence of low C3 and C4 suggests immune complex disease, the presence of low C3 and normal C4 suggests complement mediated disease. [25] See table. 1 Once the biopsy confirms the diagnosis, further work up should be pursued to identify trigger mechanism like infection, gammopathies etc. [25]

Fibrillary and immunotactoid glomerulonephritis are diagnosed by the presence of non-amyloid deposits in electron microscope. [35, 38].

Management

There is general management and specific management. Details are beyond the scope of the chapter. General management includes optimum blood pressure control, lipid management, low salt diet, and use of ACE/ARBs and diuretics when acceptable. In addition to this, the management includes management of chronic kidney disease in general, like bone and mineral disease, anemia, lipid management, vaccination, diabetic control and acid-base management. [39].

Milder forms of glomerulonephritis might require only conservative management, while severe form of glomerulonephritis will require more aggressive therapy. Therapeutic agents used include steroids in addition to immuno-modulating agents like cyclophosphamide, rituximab, mycophenolate mofetil and tacrolimus. Some of these patients require plasmapheresis and renal replacement therapy. The choice of agent is at the discretion of the nephrologist, patient comorbidities, extent and reversibility of damage and patient response.

Good pastures syndrome, fibrillary glomerulonephritis and Immunotactoid glomerulonephritis are the most difficult to treat glomerulonephritis. [38]

Patients who are chronically immunosuppressed need to have PCP prophylaxis, calcium and vitamin D supplements. The patients on chronic steroids need to be regularly screened for osteoporosis, which can be again tricky in patients with chronic kidney disease. People tend avoid bisphosphonates in the patients with GFR less than 45. [40]

Conclusion

Glomerular hematuria should be differentiated from any kind of hematuria. A detailed history and physical along with a thorough urine examination is a good starting point. The presence of certain red flags such as the presence and degree of proteinuria as well as the level of renal function should be sought by the primary care provider. If there is no proteinuria or abnormal renal function there is very limited utility in pursuing further extensive work-up, however, in the presence of aforementioned factors, early referral to nephrologist is reasonable.

The nephrologists need to go through the different causes of glomerular hematuria, order the appropriate investigations. On occasions, the nephrologist may need to start aggressive therapy even before a final diagnosis is reached as in patients who have RPGN.

References

[1]   Tiebosch ATMG, Frederick PM, Van Breda Vriesman PJC et al: Thin basement-membrane nephropathy. *N. Eng. J. Med.* 1989; 320:14-8.

[2]   Thaller TR, Wang L: Evaluation of asymptomatic microscopic hematuria in adults. *Am. Fam. Physician.* 60: 1999; 1143-1152.

[3]   Grossfeld GD, Wolf JS Jr, Litwan MS, et al: Asymptomatic microscopic hematuria in adults: Summary of the AUA best practice policy recommendations. *Am. Fam. Physician* 2001;63:1145-1154.

[4]   Cohen RA, and Brown RS: Microscopic hematuria. N Engl J Med 2003;348: 2330-8.

[5]   Schramek P, Moritsch A, Haschkowitz H, Binder BR and Maier B: In vitro generation of dysmorphic erythrocytes. *Kidney Int.* 1989;36(1):72-77.

[6]   Birch DF, Fairley KF, Whitworth JA, Forbes I, Fairley JK, Cheshire GR, Ryan GB: Urinary erythrocyte morphology in the diagnosis of glomerular hematuria. *Clin. Nephrol.*1983;20(2):78.

[7]   Davin JC. Henoch-Schönlein purpura nephritis: pathophysiology, treatment, and future strategy. *Clin. J. Am. Soc. Nephrol.* 2011;6:679-89.

[8]   D'Amico G. The commonest glomerulonephritis in the world: IgA nephropathy. *Q. J. Med.* 1987;64:709-27.

[9]   Meadow SR, Scott DG: Berger disease: Henoch-Schonlein without the rash. *J. Pediatr.* 106: 27–32, 1985.

[10] Wehbe E, Salem C, Simon JF, Navaneethan SD and Pohl M: IgA-dominant Staphylococcus infection-associated glomerulonephritis: case reports and review of the literature. *NDT Plus* (2011) 0:1–5.

[11] Boyd JK, Cheung CK, Molyneux K, Feehally J, Barratt K: An update on the pathogenesis and treatment of IgA nephropathy. *Kidney International* (2012) 81, 833–843.

[12] Berthoux F, Mohey H, Laurent B, Mar- iat C, Afiani A, Thibaudin L. Predicting the risk for dialysis or death in IgA nephropathy. *J. Am. Soc. Nephrol.* 2011;22:752- 61.

[13] Mariani AJ, Mariani MC, Macchioni C.: The significance of adult hematuria: 1,000 hematuria evaluations including a risk-benefit and cost-effectiveness analysis. *J. Urol.* 1989;141: 350-355.

[14] Vizjak A, Ferluga D: Spectrum of collagen type IV nephropathies: from thin basement membrane nephropathy to Alport syndrome. *Srp. Arh. Celok Lek.* 2008 Dec;136 Suppl 4:323-6.

[15] Jais JP, Knebelmann B, Giatras I, De Marchi M, Rizzoni G, et al: X-linked Alport syndrome: Natural history in 195 families and genotype–phenotype correlations in males. *J. Am. Soc. Nephrol.* 11: 649–657, 2000.

[16] Pochet J-M, Bobrie G, Landias P, Goldfarb B, Grunfeld J-P: Renal Prognosis in Alport's and Related Syndromes: Influence of the Mode of Inheritance Nephrol Dial Transplant 1989; 4:1016-1021. 18. Catalá López JL, Fábregas Brouard M: Acanthocyturia is more efficient in to differentiate glomerular from non-glomerular hematuria then dysmorphic erythrocytes. *Arch. Esp. Urol.* 2002 Mar;55(2):164-6.

[17] Catalá López JL, Fábregas Brouard M: Acanthocyturia is more efficient in to differentiate glomerular from non-glomerular hematuria then dysmorphic erythrocytes. *Arch. Esp. Urol.* 2002 Mar;55(2):164-6.

[18] Montseny JJ, Meyrier A, Kleinknecht D, Callard P: The current spectrum of infectious glomerulonephritis. Experience with 76 patients and review of the literature. *Medicine* (Baltimore). 1995 Mar;74(2):63-73.

[19] Wen YK: The spectrum of adult postinfectious glomerulonephritis in the new millennium. *Ren. Fail.* 2009;31(8):676-82.

[20] WG Couser: Rapidly progressive glomerulonephritis: Classification, pathogenetic mechanisms, and therapy. *Am. J. Kidney Dis.* 1988;11(6):449.

[21] Boseman P, Lewin M, Dillon J, Sethi S: Marfan syndrome, MPGN, and bacterial endocarditis. *Am. J. Kidney Dis.* 2008;51(4):697.

[22] Smith RJ, Alexander J, Barlow PN, Botto M, Cassavant TL, et al: Dense Deposit Disease Focus Group. New approaches to the treatment of dense deposit disease: *J. Am Soc Nephrol.* 2007;18(9):2447.

[23] Rennke HG: Secondary membranoproliferative glomerulonephritis. *Kidney Int.* 1995;47(2):643.

[24] Hulton SA, Risdon RA, Dillon MJ: Mesangiocapillary glomerulonephritis associated with meningococcal meningitis, C3 nephritic factor and persistently low complement C3 and C5. *Pediatr. Nephrol.* 1992;6(3):239.

[25] Sanjeev Sethi, M.D., Ph.D., and Fernando C. Fervenza, M.D., Ph.D.: Membranoproliferative Glomerulonephritis. A New Look at an Old Entity *N. Engl. J. Med.* 2012;366:1119-31.

[26] Savige J: Haematuria in asymptomatic individuals *BMJ* 2001;322:942–3.

[27] Seo P, Stone JH: The antineutrophil cytoplasmic antibody-associated vasculitides. *Am. J. Med.* 2004;117(1):39-50.

[28] Goodpasture EW: The significance of certain pulmonary lesions in relation to the etiology of influenza. *Am. J. Med. Sci* 1919; 158:863-870.

[29] Saus J, Wieslander J, Langeveld J, et al: Identification of the Goodpasture antigen as the a3(IV) chain of collagen IV. *J. Biol. Chem.* 1988; 263:13374-13380.

[30] Feehally J, Floege J, Savill J, Turner AN: Glomerular injury and glomerular response. In: Cameron JS, Davison AM, Grunfeld J-P, et al., ed. Oxford Textbook of Nephrology, 3rd ed. Oxford: *Oxford University Press*; 2005:363-388.

[31] Appel GB, Waldman M: Update on the treatment of lupus nephritis. *Kidney Int* 2006; 70:1403-1412.

[32] Weening JJ, D'Agati VD, Schwartz MM, Seshan SV, Alpers CE, Appel GB, et al: International Society of Nephrology Working Group on the Classification of Lupus Nephritis, Renal Pathology Society Working Group on the Classification of Lupus Nephritis: The classification of glomerulonephritis in systemic lupus erythematosus revisited. *Kidney Int.* 2004;65(2):521.

[33] Jennette JC: Rapidly progressive crescentic glomerulonephritis. *Kidney Int* 2003; 63:1164-1177.

[34] Duna GF, Galperin C, Hoffman GS: Wegener's granulomatosis. *Rheum. Dis. Clin. North. Am.* 1995; 21:949-986.

[35] Nasr SH; Valeri AM; Cornell LD; Fidler ME; Sethi S; Leung N; Fervenza FC: Fibrillary glomerulonephritis: a report of 66 cases from a single institution. *Clin. J. Am. Soc. Nephrol.* 2011; 6(4):775.

[36] Sokolosky MC: Hematuria. Emerg. *Med. Clin. North Am.* 2001;19: 621-632.

[37] Wen YK, Chen ML: The significance of atypical morphology in the changes of spectrum of postinfectious glomerulonephritis. *Clin. Nephrol.* 2010 Mar;73(3):173-9.

[38] Rosenstock JL, Markowitz GS, Valeri AM, Sacchi G, Appel GB, D'Agati VD: Fibrillary and immunotactoid glomerulonephritis: Distinct entities with different clinical and pathologic features. *Kidney Int.* 2003 Apr;63(4):1450-61.

[39] KDIGO 2012 Clinical Practice Guideline for the Evaluation and Management of Chronic Kidney disease. *Kid. Intern. Supplements* 2013; 3(1).

[40] Miller PD: Is There a Role for Bisphosphonates in Chronic Kidney Disease? *Seminars in Dialysis—Vol 20*, No 3 (May–June) 2007 pp. 186–190.

In: Hematuria
Editors: Nikhil Vasdev and G. Boustead

ISBN: 978-1-63463-073-3
© 2015 Nova Science Publishers, Inc.

Chapter 7

Hematuria: Diagnosis and Management

Nilum Rajora * *and Ramesh Saxena*
Internal Medicine, Division of Nephrology,
University of Texas Southwestern Medical Center, Dallas, Texas, US

Introduction

Hematuria is defined as the presence of red blood cells (RBC) in the urine. It can be gross hematuria, visible to naked eyes, or microscopic hematuria. Either of these can be from benign or more serious causes like malignancy. Patients with gross hematuria present earlier due to concern about change in urine color, while it may be an incidental finding among patients with microscopic hematuria. Patient's medical history and presenting symptoms assist in further evaluation and management of the patients with hematuria. In this chapter we will review the prevalence, clinical presentation, etiology, evaluation and management of hematuria in adults.

Prevalence of Hematuria

Prevalence of hematuria varies in adults depending on the age, gender, frequency of testing, and presence of risk factors. In general population, prevalence of microscopic hematuria ranges from 0.19% to 16% and gross hematuria can occur in up to 2.5% of the population. Transient hematuria can be seen in 6-40% of the population. The prevalence of hematuria is as high as 21% among older men with risk of urological disease. Presence of underlying abnormality of genitourinary tract does not differ among patients with persistent or intermittent hematuria.

* (Phone): 214-645-6401. (Fax): 214-648-2071. Email: Nilum.rajora@utsouthwestern.edu.

Clinical Presentation

Presence of even small amount of blood in urine (1ml/1L urine) can change the color of urine to be visible to the patients. Besides the presence of gross blood in urine, myoglobinuria or hemoglobinuria can also cause brown discoloration of the urine and result in a positive test for blood by dipstick analysis of urine. However, they can be differentiated form hematuria by absence of red blood cells on microscopic analysis of urine. This chapter will focus only on hematuria.

Hematuria can be gross or microscopic, and clinical presentation depends on the underlying etiology. Most of the patients with gross hematuria present early with the concerns of change in urine color.

It may cause anxiety and concern among the patients and family members. If patient has persistent gross hematuria, it can present with iron deficiency anemia and hemodynamic instability with signs of organ hypoperfusion, including dizziness and hypotension. Patients with gross hematuria can also develop obstructive nephropathy from the clot and present with supra-pubic fullness, pain, acute kidney injury and urinary retention. Recurring gross hematuria can occur among patients with nephrolithiasis, pyelonephritis or cystic renal disease. These patients present with acute or chronic flank pain. Hematuria associated with malignancy may also present with tumor-associated malaise, weight loss, pains and night sweats.

Patients with microscopic hematuria may have transient or persistent hematuria. It can be an isolated and incidental finding on urine analysis or can be associated with systemic disease. Patient with microscopic hematuria associated with nephrolithiasis or urinary tract infection, present with renal colic or dysuria and fever respectively. Glomerular Hematuria can be isolated or associated with proteinuria. Patients with isolated hematuria of glomerular origin are usually asymptomatic.

If microscopic hematuria is associated with proteinuria patients may present with manifestations of renal disease like hypertension, edema, renal insufficiency and uremia. Patients with hematuria associated with collagen vascular disease present with other systemic manifestations of skin rash, joint pain and fever.

Etiology

Blood in urine can originate from any location along the urinary tract. Hematuria can be of benign cause like vigorous exercise prior to urine analysis or can be from more serious etiologies like bladder cancer or renal cell carcinoma. Complete list of causes of hematuria are listed in Table 1. Gross (visible to naked eyes) or microscopic hematuria can originate from similar or different etiologies as discussed below.

- **Gross Hematuria:** Majority of the patients with gross hematuria present early in the disease process due to concern about discoloration of the urine. Common causes of gross hematuria are nephrolithiasis, infections and malignancy of urinary tract. Urological malignancies include transitional cell carcinoma of the bladder, renal cell carcinoma; and ureteric, prostate or urethral malignancy. Occasionally, gross hematuria may ensue after kidney biopsy. Some of the benign causes of gross hematuria include urinary tract infection (UTI), benign prostate hyperplasia (BPH) or trauma from catheterization. Recurring gross hematuria can occur with nephrolithiasis, pyelonephritis or cystic renal disease and may present with chronic pain.

- *Microscopic Hematuria:* Microscopic hematuria can be isolated or can be associated with proteinuria. Microscopic hematuria without proteinuria is often an incidental finding. It can be transient or persistent. Transient hematuria is usually associated with benign causes like vigorous activity, contamination with menstrual blood or urethral irritation. Persistent hematuria can originate from renal or extra renal sources. Hematuria associated with proteinuria, dysmorphic RBCs, RBC casts and renal insufficiency are of glomerular origin. Extra-renal sources of microscopic hematuria include genitourinary tract i.e., ureter, bladder and urethra. Complete list of causes of hematuria are listed in Table 1.

Table 1. Causes of Hematuria

1.	Renal	2.	Extra Renal
a.	**Glomerular**	a.	**Ureter**
	IgA nephropathy		Ureteral Stone
	Alport's Syndrome		Ureteral malignancy
	Thin basement membrane disease	b.	**Bladder**
	Lupus nephritis		Bladder Malignancy
	Post infectious GN		Cystitis
	Membranoproliferative GN		Trauma
	FSGS		Parasitic Infection
	Crescentic GN	c.	**Prostate**
b.	**Tubulointerstitial**		Benign Prostate Hyperplasia
	Acute Interstitial Nephritis		Prostate Cancer
	Chronic interstitial Nephritis		Prostatitis
	Nephrolithiasis	d.	**Urethra**
c.	**Other**		UTI
	Renal Infarction		Urethritis
	Cystic Renal Disease		Trauma
	Renal Vein thrombosis		Sexually Transmitted Disease

Hematuria can originate anywhere in the urinary tract. It can be or renal or extra-renal origin and have different etiologies as discussed below.

1. Renal: Hematuria can be of glomerular or non-glomerular origin. These can be differentiated based on the clinical history, urine analysis and renal function.
   - Glomerular: Isolated glomerular hematuria, without significant proteinuria, is usually asymptomatic and is an incidental finding. Urine with red blood cell casts, dysmorphic red blood cells, and proteinuria suggest hematuria of glomerular origin. Usually, degree of hematuria does not have a correlation with extent of renal damage, unlike amount of proteinuria which correlates with

degree of the renal disease. Most common cause of isolated glomerular hematuria is IgA nephropathy [1]. Other causes of isolated hematuria include thin basement membrane disease and Alport Syndrome. Microscopic hematuria associated with proteinuria is seen from different causes of glomerulonephritis (GN) e.g., Lupus nephritis, Post infectious GN, focal segmental glomerulosclerosis (FSGS), crescentic GN and membranoproliferative GN. See Table 1 for complete list.

- Tubulointerstitial: Microscopic, and occasionally gross hematuria can be seen with drug induced acute interstitial nephritis (AIN) in less than 50% of cases [2]. Hematuria is more common with methicillin and other β-lactam class of antibiotics [3]. Up to 90% of the patients with AIN from β-lactam class of antibiotics develop hematuria. Clindamycin associated AIN can also present with gross hematuria (up to 8.3% of the patients) and the incidence of hematuria can vary from 3.5% to 62.5% among patients with acute kidney injury (AKI) [4].

- Other renal causes: Other causes of microscopic hematuria include nephrolithiasis, cystic renal disease, pyelonephritis, papillary necrosis, renal infarctions, vasculitis, renal arterial emboli or thrombosis, renal vein thrombosis, loin pain hematuria and bleeding diathesis.

2. Extrarenal: More than 60% of the cases of hematuria are from extra-renal source. Whereas some cases stem from benign such as benign prostate hyperplasia, infection and trauma from catheterization, others can be from more serious etiologies like prostate, bladder or urinary tract malignancies. Different etiologies based on the location of origin of hematuria are listed below.

- Ureter: Ureteral causes of hematuria include ureteral stone or ureteral malignancy.

- Bladder: Bladder cancer is the most common cause of gross hematuria. The incidence of bladder malignancy in high risk patients ranges from 5% (persistent microscopic hematuria) to > 20% (with gross hematuria). Other etiologies of hematuria of bladder origin include cystitis, catheter trauma, stones, drugs (like cyclophosphamide) and parasitic infections (such as schistosomaisis).

- Urethra: Hematuria of urethral origin presents with blood in urine at the beginning of urination. Hematuria usually clears by the end of urination indicating origin of hematuria from more distal site of genitourinary tract. Urinary tract infection, urethritis, catheter trauma or sexually transmitted diseases can present with hematuria of urethral origin.

- Prostate: Benign prostate hyperplasia, prostate cancer and prostatitis can present with isolated hematuria.

Emergent Causes of Hematuria

Some of the causes of hematuria may require immediate attention due to likelihood of poor outcome without immediate care and should be considered in initial evaluation. These include abdominal aortic aneurysm dissection, renal infarction, urogenital trauma, and bladder outlet obstruction from the clots (Table 2).

Table 2. Emergent Causes of Hematuria

Aortic Aneurysm Rupture
Renal Infarction
Genitourinary Trauma/ Post kidney biopsy persistent hematuria
Bladder Outlet Obstruction from blood clot
Bleeding diathesis
Rapidly progressive glomerulonephritis
Nephrolithiasis causing obstruction
Hemorrhagic Cystitis

Signs and Symptoms

Signs and symptoms of hematuria depend on the underlying cause of hematuria (Table 3). Hematuria related to cystitis, UTI or pyelonephritis usually causes fever, urinary urgency, dysuria, and urinary frequency or flank pain. Patients with nephrolithiasis develop colicky pain and gross or microscopic hematuria. Patients with malignancy related hematuria may also develop other signs and symptoms of malignancy like weight loss, malaise, night sweats and pain. Hematuria associated with polycystic kidney disease can be associated with flank pain, abdominal fullness and abdominal distention related to cysts. If gross hematuria is of significant amount, it can cause hemodynamic compromise with poor organ perfusion. Isolated hematuria of glomerular origin is usually asymptomatic but patients with hematuria associated with proteinuria and renal disease may develop hypertension, volume overload or uremia.

Table 3.

Etiology of Hematuria	Signs and Symptoms
Urinary Tract Infections	Fever, chills, dysuria, increased urinary frequency
Nephrolithiasis	Colicky abdominal pain with radiation to groin
Genito-urinary malignancies	Weight loss, gross or microscopic hematuria, malaise, pain
Cystic kidney diseases	Flank pain and fullness
Glomerular diseases	hypertension, Edema and foamy urine if associated with proteinuria
Aortic aneurysm rupture, hemorrhagic cystitis or persistent gross hematuria	Hypotension, cardiovascular collapse, anemia
Autoimmune	Rashes, joint pain, renal insufficiency

Pathophysiology

Normal individuals can excrete upto 10^5 red blood cells in the urine every day and is not considered pathogenic. Presence of more than 2-3 RBCs/ high power field (HPF) is of clinical significance. Hematuria can result from injury to the kidney or to another site in the urinary tract. It can be localized to the injury site or can be the manifestation of systemic disorder like bleeding diathesis, autoimmune disorders (Lupus, Goodpasture syndrome). Hematuria from non-glomerular causes is related to the bleeding from the urinary tract either by direct injury to the urogenital tract or bleeding from the malignant growth.

Glomerular hematuria is usually from damage of filtration barrier. The glomerular filtration barrier consists of three major components: glomerular endothelial cell, the basement membrane and visceral epithelial cell (podocyte). This provides a selective barrier to bigger molecules while allowing conductance of small and midsize molecules from the plasma. Alteration or damage to glomerular basement membrane (GBM) can cause leakage of the blood cells in the urinary space as seen in Alport Syndrome, IgA nephropathy or Thin Basement Membrane Disease. Damage to other components of filtration barrier (endothelial cells, podocytes) can cause combination of hematuria and proteinuria. As the RBCs have to transit through the urinary tract, they undergo osmotic and chemical stress, causing change in their shape. Precipitation of Tamm-Horsfall muco-protein secreted by renal tubular cells or presence of proteinuria along with RBCs can cause the formation of RBC casts and is pathological findings of GN. Thus, urine analysis with dysmorphic RBCs, RBC casts and proteinuria suggest hematuria of glomerular origin.

Transient hematuria is usually benign finding. It can occur from contamination of menstrual blood in the urine or after vigorous exercise. Vigorous exercise can cause injury to GU tract causing transient hematuria. Repeat urine analysis, in absence of active menstruation or recent vigorous activity, shows absence of blood or RBCs in the urine.

Work Up

Microscopic hematuria is usually of benign significance in the majority of the patients. A detailed history and physical exam is essential part of evaluation for hematuria. Recent history of vigorous exercise, menstruation and sexual activity usually suggest benign cause of isolated hematuria and can be confirmed by absence of hematuria on repeat urine analysis (UA). Repeat UA can be performed after completion of menstruation and absence of vigorous activity within 24 hours of earlier UA. Persistent hematuria requires further evaluation (Figure 1). Work up of persistent hematuria involves UA, urine cytology and radiological imaging, as indicated. Complete guideline for work up of hematuria is outlined in Figure 1and is discussed more in details below.

a. Clinical History: Detailed history of patient with hematuria includes timing of hematuria, menstruation, urinary frequency, and urinary hesitancy, association with pain, history of anticoagulation and change in weight. Urinary hesitancy and urgency may require GU work up while colicky abdominal pain may prompt evaluation for nephrolithiasis. Coagulopathy should be ruled out in patient on anticoagulation.

b. Physical Exam: Patient should have blood pressure checked to evaluate for GN or hypertensive emergency leading to hematuria. Prostate and genitourinary exam should be performed to examine for prostatic lesions such as BPH, prostatitis or prostate cancer. External urethral exam should be performed for presence of any lesions. Signs and symptoms of autoimmune diseases include skin rashes, join pains or join swelling. Patients with Alport syndrome can have deafness and should be evaluated for any hearing loss.

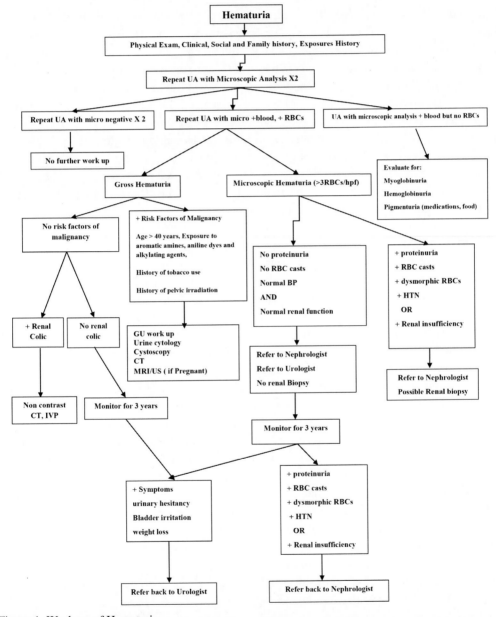

Figure 1. Work up of Hematuria.

c. Urine Analysis: Routine screening for microscopic hematuria for bladder cancer is not recommended by American Urological Association [5] and other international societies [6]. Majority of the patients are identified with hematuria in routine laboratory work up. If a patient has an incidental finding of microscopic hematuria on UA then repeat, clean catch, mid-stream urine specimen should be sent to confirm hematuria. If routine dipstick urine analysis is positive for blood then microscopic urine analysis should be performed for urinary sediments and presence of RBC. Positive dipstick test but negative microscopy should be repeated with three additional urine samples as many factors can cause false negative and false positive urine analysis. False positive UA can be seen from myoglobin, hemoglobin, and menstrual blood. False negative UA can result from delay in analyzing urine sample, vitamin C ingestion and urine pH <5.1. Transient microscopic hematuria is benign and does not require further work up. Transient microscopic hematuria can occur in 6-39% of the general population from vigorous exercise, sexual intercourse, mild trauma or menstrual contamination. If the patient has three negative UA then no further work up is required.

Presence of pyuria and other clinical signs and symptoms indicate UTI and should be treated with appropriate antibiotics. After the treatment of UTI, repeat urine analysis should be performed in 6 weeks. Hematuria associated with presence of proteinuria and dysmorphic RBC cells or RBC casts on microscopic exam indicates hematuria of glomerular origin and requires nephrology evaluation for renal parenchymal disease. Isolated glomerular hematuria without any proteinuria or renal insufficiency can be monitored as outpatient, without renal biopsy, while hematuria associated with proteinuria and renal insufficiency may require renal biopsy to determine the etiology of renal disease.

d. Urological evaluation: Presence of gross hematuria or microscopic hematuria with risk factors of malignancy requires urological work up. Risk factors for genitourinary (GU) malignancies include age greater than 40 years, exposure to aromatic amines, aniline dyes and alkylating chemotherapeutic agents, history of tobacco use, and pelvic irradiation. Patients with risk factors for urogenital cancer should be referred for urological work up which includes diagnostic cystoscopy, urine cytology and cytology of bladder washings. If indicated, patients may require imaging with excretory urography for upper urinary tract imaging; renal ultrasound or contrast enhanced computerized tomography to evaluate for renal or ureteral mass, renal calculi or cystic disease.

Recent guidelines from American Urological Association (AUA) were published for diagnosis, evaluation and follow up of asymptomatic hematuria in adults [7].According to these guidelines, all patients aged older than 35 years with micro or macroscopic hematuria should get cystoscopy. As the probability of genitourinary (GU) malignancy is low in younger age group, indication for cystoscopy can be determined based on the clinical history in patients younger than 35 years. However, any patient with risk factors for GU malignancy should undergo cystoscopy, regardless of the age [7]. Cystoscopy provides the direct visualization and biopsy of bladder mucosa and bladder lesions.

e. Laboratory Data: According to AUA guidelines, patients with asymptomatic microscopic hematuria should have renal function checked prior to imaging studies which might involve exposure to IV contrast. Presence of glomerular hematuria requires simultaneous renal and urological evaluation. Presence of proteinuria and renal insufficiency may require glomerulonephritis work up.

f. Radiological Imaging: Several radiological imaging are available for evaluation of GU tract. Among them, three imaging modalities are commonly employed; ultrasonography (US), intravenous urography (IVP), and multiphasic computed tomography urography. For complete evaluation of renal parenchyma, excretory urography should be supplemented with renal ultrasound. Ultrasound has a limited role in the detection of renal calculi but is recommended by the European Society of Urogenital Radiology (ESUR) guidelines for the investigation of painless hematuria. Ultrasound is the test of choice for evaluation of internal architecture of cystic renal masses and determining Bosniak grades of a renal mass but the sensitivity of ultrasound for detecting renal lesions less than 1 cm is only 26%.

Ideal imaging study for work up of hematuria should have minimal risk to the patient while providing the appropriate evaluation of the GU tract. According to American College of Radiology, multiphasic computed tomography urography (CTU) is the best imaging modality to work up hematuria. Inclusion of high resolution imaging during excretory phase allows most sensitive and specific imaging for detecting lesions of renal parenchyma and upper GU tract. Prior to administration of iodinated contrast, renal function should be checked to avoid contrast induced nephropathy. AUA guidelines also recommend multiphasic CTU over ultrasound + IVP for work up of hematuria. Magnetic resonance imaging is an acceptable alternative for patients who have contraindications to CTU like pregnancy, allergy to contrast and renal insufficiency. Some patients may not be able to get MRI due to presence of metal in the body. Use of IV contrast, Gadolinium, for MRI should be avoided in patients with chronic kidney disease with GFR <30ml/min/1.75M2 due to risk of developing nephrogenic systemic fibrosis (NSF). Patients with relative contraindications for CT and MRI who need evaluation of the collecting system can be evaluated with non-contrast CT or renal ultrasound with retrograde pyelogram.

According to the ESUR guidelines, patient's imaging modality should be chosen based on the risk factors of the patients [8]. Patients with low risk of malignancy can be evaluated with ultrasound and cystoscopy. Medium-risk patients require ultrasound and cystoscopy and if those tests are negative, excretory urography or CT urography should be performed. High-risk patients should have CT urography and cystoscopy for thorough renal and urinary tract imaging.

Evaluation for possible nephrolithiasis includes non-contrast helical CT scan, intravenous pyelography (IVP), abdominal plain film, and ultrasonography. Non-contrast CT with 3-5 mm thickness cuts is gold standard for work up of nephrolithiasis. It is about 97% specific and 60% sensitive for detection of renal calculi. Radiolucent stones like Indinavir, uric acid and cysteine stones may not be detected on routine radiological imaging and require contrast enhanced imaging.

Pregnant patients with microscopic hematuria can be evaluated with renal U/S and MRI as likelihood of malignancy is low in this population and other work up can be done after the delivery.

g. Urine Cytology: Urine cytology is specific but not highly sensitive test for screening of bladder cancer and is currently not recommended for routine evaluation. Negative urine cytology does not preclude GU malignancy and does not replace full work up. Sensitivity of urine cytology can be increased by using first morning void sample and can be considered in patients with positive risk factors for GU malignancy. Other urine tumor markers for bladder cancer screening are studied and include; bladder tumor antigen, carcinoembryonic antigen, nuclear matrix protein 22 and Lewis X antigen. These tumor markers are currently not available for screening of bladder cancer.

Management

Patients with microscopic hematuria with normal renal function can be evaluated in non-emergent setting and work up is outlined in Figure 1. Even the most serious cases of gross hematuria may not require hospital admission as most of the cases are not immediately life threatening and can be managed with blood transfusions and transurethral procedures. Any patient with gross hematuria should be assessed for hemodynamic stability prior to any work up. Clinical examination of the patient with gross hematuria should include assessment of cardiovascular status, bladder exam for palpable mass or urinary retention, genital exam for external lesions and digital rectal exam for BPH or prostate masses. If patient shows signs of hemodynamic instability, appropriate supportive care should include colloids, crystalloids or vasopressors as needed. Laboratory studies should include complete blood count and renal function assessment. Patients with hemodynamic instability and gross hematuria, coagulation profile (prothrombin time, partial thromboplastin time and international normalized ratio) should be assessed and typing and cross matching for blood products should also be done. Coagulopathy should be reversed and urologist or interventional radiologist should be consulted in hemodynamically unstable patient to attain hemostasis. In a patient with gross hematuria, free drainage of urine should be ascertained. Clot formation can cause urinary retention and should be addressed immediately to avoid acute kidney injury. If urinary retention due to blood clot is present, three-way indwelling catheter should be placed to allow bladder irrigation to assist with clot removal. Patients without hemodynamic instability, urinary retention or acute kidney injury can be safely worked up as outpatient, as outlined in work up section above. Specific treatment of hematuria depends on the underlying etiology of hematuria. Asymptomatic isolated hematuria, without any concerns of malignancy or GN, does not require any treatment. Patients with abnormal laboratory or imaging studies should be treated for primary disease process. Patients with anatomical abnormalities, malignancy, and obstructive nephrolithiasis may need surgical intervention.

Follow Up

About 10% of the patients with hematuria have negative urological work up. However, patients with negative initial evaluation may still be at risk for malignancy, nephrolithiasis, mycobacterial infections, and glomerulonephritis, and therefore, require regular monitoring. As incidence of urological malignancy increases with advanced age and presence of risk factors, high-risk patients should be followed closely for about 3 years. Most malignancies will be detected by 3 years.

Follow up of the patients with hematuria includes clinical history and physical exam along with urine analysis, blood pressure check, and urine cytology. Frequency of the monitoring should be at 6, 12, 24 and 36 months [9]. If patient has urine analysis negative for hematuria for two consecutive years, then no further follow up is required. If patient develops any irritative voiding symptoms in absence of infection, or have abnormal urine cytology, then the patient should be referred to urology for repeat evaluation including cystoscopy, cytology or repeat imaging to rule out bladder cancer. Some experts suggest repeating urological work up, in high risk patients, in 2-5 years.

Patients who develop proteinuria, hypertension, dysmorphic RBCs and RBC casts in urine should be referred back to nephrologist for work up and management of possible glomerulonephritis.

Prognosis

In majority of the patients, hematuria originates from lower urinary tract. Most common benign causes of hematuria are infections and nephrolithiasis with the frequency of 20% and 25% respectively. Outcome of these patients depend on the underlying causes of infection or nephrolithiasis. Only 10% of the patients with hematuria have glomerular causes of hematuria.

Malignancy has been shown to be the most common cause of hematuria in elderly. Persistent hematuria in older patients, therefore, raises the possibility of malignancy. The risk of malignancy ranges from 0-3% in 2-5 years after initial presentation in patients with persistent hematuria. Urinary tract malignancies are more common in men than women with the ration of 2 to 1. Gross hematuria is associated with higher likelihood (22% or more) of malignancy. Among these patients, bladder cancer is the most common malignancy (9%) associated with hematuria.

Key Points

1. Hematuria is a common manifestation of diseases of kidney and urinary tract and is usually an incidental finding on urine analysis. It can be either benign or presenting sign of malignancy especially in elderly or high risk patient.
2. Myoglobinuria or hemoglobinuria can also cause brown discoloration of the urine and a positive test for blood by dipstick analysis of urine, but can be differentiated form hematuria by absence of red blood cells on microscopic analysis of urine.
3. Transient hematuria can be confirmed by absence of hematuria of repeat urine analysis and does not require any further work up.
4. Persistent hematuria requires further evaluation including urine analysis, urine cytology and radiological imaging as indicated.
5. Specific treatment of hematuria depends on the underlying etiology. Some of the causes of hematuria may require immediate attention if associated with hemodynamic compromise or obstruction. Asymptomatic isolated hematuria, without any concerns of malignancy or glomerulonephritis, does not require any treatment. Patients with abnormal laboratory or imaging studies should be treated for primary disease process. Patients with anatomical abnormalities, malignancy, and obstructive nephrolithiasis may need surgical intervention.
6. Follow up of the patients with hematuria includes clinical history and physical exam along with urine analysis, blood pressure check, and urine cytology. If patient has negative urine analysis for hematuria in two consecutive years, then no further follow up is required. If patient develops any irritative voiding symptoms in absence of

infection, or have abnormal urine cytology, then the patient should be referred back to urologist for repeat evaluation including cystoscopy, cytology or repeat imaging.

7. Patients who develop proteinuria, hypertension, dysmorphic RBCs and RBC casts in urine should be referred back to nephrologist for work up and management of possible glomerulonephritis.

References

[1]   Wyatt, R. J. & Julian, B. A. IgA nephropathy. *The New England journal of medicine* 368, 2402-2414, doi:10.1056/NEJMra1206793 (2013).

[2]   Perazella, M. A. & Markowitz, G. S. Drug-induced acute interstitial nephritis. *Nature reviews. Nephrology* 6, 461-470, doi:10.1038/nrneph.2010.71 (2010).

[3]   Rossert, J. Drug-induced acute interstitial nephritis. *Kidney international* 60, 804-817, doi:10.1046/j.1523-1755.2001.060002804.x (2001).

[4]   Xie, H. et al. Clindamycin-induced acute kidney injury: large biopsy case series. *American journal of nephrology* 38, 179-183, doi:10.1159/000354088 (2013).

[5]   Loo, R., Whittaker, J. & Rabrenivich, V. National practice recommendations for hematuria: how to evaluate in the absence of strong evidence? *The Permanente journal* 13, 37-46 (2009).

[6]   Higashihara, E. et al. Hematuria: definition and screening test methods. *International journal of urology: official journal of the Japanese Urological Association* 15, 281-284, doi:10.1111/j.1442-2042.2008.02009.x (2008).

[7]   Davis, R. et al. Diagnosis, evaluation and follow-up of asymptomatic microhematuria (AMH) in adults: AUA guideline. *The Journal of urology* 188, 2473-2481, doi:10.1016/j.juro.2012.09.078 (2012).

[8]   Van Der Molen, A. J. et al. CT urography: definition, indications and techniques. A guideline for clinical practice. *European radiology* 18, 4-17, doi:10.1007/s00330-007-0792-x (2008).

[9]   Grossfeld, G. D. et al. Evaluation of asymptomatic microscopic hematuria in adults: the American Urological Association best practice policy--part I: definition, detection, prevalence, and etiology. *Urology* 57, 599-603 (2001).

In: Hematuria
Editors: Nikhil Vasdev and G. Boustead

ISBN: 978-1-63463-073-3
© 2015 Nova Science Publishers, Inc.

Chapter 8

The Role of Screening in Patients with Hematuria

Takahiro Hirayama, Kazumasa Matsumoto, Morihiro Nishi,
Tetsuo Fujita and Masatsugu Iwamura*
Department of Urology, KITASATO University School of Medicine,
Sagamihara, Kanagawa, Japan

Keywords: Hematuria, Bladder cancer, Urothelial carcinoma

Introduction

Hematuria, both microscopic and macroscopic, is one of the main or an accompanying symptom for which patients require medical consultation or treatment in urology. Microscopic hematuria has usually been confirmed in consecutive centrifuged urine specimens with microscopy for three and more red blood cells per high-power field [1]. In population based studies, the prevalence of microscopic hematuria varied from 0.19% to 21.0% [2, 3]. Macroscopic hematuria is visible status without microscopy. The prevalence of this condition was approximately 2.5% [4]. In American Urological Association guideline, microscopic hematuria is defined as a single positive urinalysis [5]. According to redefining microscopic hematuria base on finding of a single urinalysis, the eligible patients requiring further examination would have potentially increased more than 30% [6]. The causes of hematuria can originate from the genitourinary tract, including benign prostate hyperplasia, urinary tract infection, stones, glomerular disease, trauma and urological malignancies [3, 7]. Khadra et al. reviewed 1930 patients with hematuria, in 252 of patients (13%) were found urological malignancies [8]. Thus, once hematuria was occurred, neoplasms of the

---
* Corresponding author: Takahiro HIRAYAMA, Department of Urology, KITASATO University School of Medicine, 1-15-1, Kitasato, Minami-ku, Sagamihara, Kanagawa, 252-0374, Japan, Tel.: +081-42-778-9091, Fax: +081-42-778-9374, E-mail: thirayam@med.kitasato-u.ac.jp.

genitourinary tract need to be ruled out in the patients with hematuria, even if those have been excluded benign diseases before [9].

Investigations

Hematuria Screening

In a population based study, red blood cells were found in the urine of 13% asymptomatic adults [10]. Urinary dipsticks have been useful for detecting asymptomatic microscopic hematuria. As this testing is simple and inexpensive, it is so popular among primary care physicians [11]. Sensitivity of the testing is up to 100%, but specificity ranges from 65% to 99% [12]. A positive result is simply a color change due to oxidation of a test-strip reagent. False-positive results on dipstick analyses are possibly due to myoglobinuria, hemoglobinuria, concentrated urine, or oxidizing contaminations in the urine. Thus, an initial finding of microscopic hematuria on urinary dipstick should be confirmed using microscopic evaluation of the urinary sediment.

Table 1. Risk factors for significant disease in patients with microscopic hematuria

Smoking history
Occupational exposure to chemicals or dyes (benzenes or aromatic amines)
History of macrohematuria
Age >40 years
History of urologic disorder or disease
History of irritative vioiding symptoms
History of urinary tract infection
Analgesic abuse
History of pelvic irradiation

Britton et al. investigated the ability of urine dipsticks to detect early bladder cancer in a group of men in the community [13]. In 2356 men more than 60 years old, the urine was tested with a dipstick for the presence of blood. A total of 474 men (20.1%) had dipstick hematuria including 17 men (3.4%) with bladder cancer. Khadra et al. reported that 92 (9.4%) of 982 patients with microscopic hematuria were found urological malignancies in their prospective study [8]. Thompson et al. reviewed the results of routine urologic evaluation of microscopic hematuria [14]. Of 2005 men, 85 (4%) had asymptomatic microscopic hematuria and subsequently underwent urologic investigations. Only one of these 85 patients had bladder cancer.

As the risk of significant disease in a patient with microscopic hematuria but without symptom is low, the evaluation for those patients can be costly. It is important to determine which patients require urologic studies. Risk factors can help in determining which patients are at higher risk of urinary tract and bladder cancer (Table1) [3].

Microscopic hematuria is commonly encountered in patients taking anticoagulant drugs. It has been shown that up to 40% of patients on anticoagulant therapy have microscopic hematuria [15]. Current recommended anticoagulation schedules do not predispose patients to hematuria [16]. The likelihood of finding cancer in the anticoagulated patients with hematuria was no different from that in the overall group [8]. The decision to evaluate a patient with hematuria should not be based on the fact on having anticoagulants.

Urine Cytology

Voided urinary cytology is recommended in all patients who have risk factors of urothelial cancer (Table 1) [3]. Sensitivity of cytology varied from 26% to 67% and specificity ranged from 82% to 97% [8, 17]. Washing urine samples may improve sensitivity. If malignant or atypical cells are identified, cytstoscopy is required. Although cytology has an acceptable sensitivity for high grade carcinoma and carcinoma in situ, it is less sensitive for low grade carcinoma or upper urinary tract carcinoma [3, 17]. In the study by Khadra et al., of 1930 patients 14 were diagnosed with upper urinary tract carcinomas without positive with cytology. However, of 230 patients who diagnosed with bladder cancer 61 patients showed positive cytology in the same study [8]. As cytology does not completely exclude urological malignancies, if microscopic hematuria would continue in patients with negative cytology, cystoscopy also should be considered.

Cystoscopy

Studies have shown that the sensitivity of cystoscopy for bladder cancer is between 66% and 79%, with the specificity between 95% and 100% [19]. Cystoscopy with a rigid or a flexible cystoscope can be performed under local anesthesia. The tissue can be taken from suspicious lesions for further analysis during the procedure, but this modality is relatively invasive. Compared with flexible cystoscopy, rigid cystoscopy causes more pain so that it can be occasionally performed under anesthesia in male patients. Although rigid cystoscopy has been widely used, it can be sometimes difficult to detect tumors at the anterior bladder neck. While flexible cystoscopy may be overcome this problem, but it was not completely painless during the procedure without anesthesia.

Cystoscopy is recommended in all patients with risk factors for bladder cancer. Even if patients with risk factors are younger than 40 years, cystoscopy should be considered. In patients younger than 40 years with no risk for bladder cancer, cystoscopy may be deferred, but cytology should be performed [20].

Ultrasound

In patients with hematuria, ultrasound can be useful to detect renal cell carcinoma, bladder cancer, upper urinary tract urothelial carcinoma, and benign diseases including hydronephrosis and urolithiasis [3]. It also can assess the prostate gland and the estimation of residual urine volume. As ultrasound does not have the risk of radiation exposure or the allergy of contrast media, it can be safely performed in pregnant women and children.

However, ultrasound has a lower diagnostic yield. It has an approximately 40% sensitivity for identifying renal tumors, and is less sensitive for upper urinary tract urothelial carcinoma because sound waves cannot penetrate deeply [19]. Limitations remain this procedure, for example the detection of small lesions and the depending on the expertise of operator.

Radiographic Investigations

Intravenous pyelography (IVP) is used to be performed as an initial radiographic study [3, 8].

The purpose of the study is to obtain an anatomical and functional evaluation of the urinary tract. IVP by itself has limited sensitivity in detecting urological malignancies, however, ultrasound needs to be combined to improve sensitivity [8].

Recently, computed tomography (CT) urography with intravenous contrast has been considered as the best imaging modality for the evaluation. Especially, multi-phasic CT urography including sufficient and excretory phases is the best imaging modality of choice because it has the highest sensitivity and specificity for the imaging the upper urinary tracts [3]. Helical CT with urography is preferred if technology is available [21]. CT urography has been shown to find more than 40% of hematuria-causing lesions missed by other studies [21]. Sensitivity in patients with hematuria varies from 94.1% to 100%, with approximately 97% specificity [21, 22].

Plain film abdominal radiography can be performed at the end of the CT examination to assess the upper urinary tract and bladder, likely to have the image of IVP. It is well known that the use of iodinated contrast may cause acute renal failure so that an estimated of renal function, including estimated glomerular filtration rate (eGFR), serum creatinine and blood urea nitrogen (BUN), should be obtained to assess preexisting renal dysfunction before the examination.

However, the incidence of death after the intravenous administration of contrast media has been reported to be one case per 40,000 contrast material injections [23]. In patients with renal insufficiency, the allergy of contrast media or pregnancy, alternative modalities including magnetic resonance urography (MRU), retrograde pyelography, ultrasound and these combinations should be considered.

Biological Markers

Recently, voided urinary markers have been examined for the early detection of bladder cancer. A recent study showed a panel of microRNAs with a high sensitivity for bladder cancer [24].

Applied to patients with hematuria, the panel would be found 94% of urothelial cancers and reduced the necessity of cystscopy to 26%. Proteomics analyses which can facilitate large-scale quantitative comparisons of protein expression also have been developed. The analyses of unknown proteins and functions may enhance the preferential markers and offer a better way to screen for bladder cancer [25].

Using recent advances in molecular techniques, biological markers potentially have an important role in screening for and monitoring of bladder cancers.

Long-Term Outcome in Patients with Negative Study for Hematuria

The frequency of serious urological disease in patients with asymptomatic microscopic hematuria is low ranged from 0.5% to 5.0% [7, 10]. According to previous study, more than 60% of patients with hematuria (1168/1930 patients) were no disease after evaluating whole urinary tract, and were not observed a subsequent or de novo neoplastic disease during follow-up ranged 2.5 to 4.2 years [8]. Madeb at al. reported 14-year outcomes of 234 men aged more than 50 years with microscopic hematuria [26]. Two of 234 men (0.85%) developed bladder cancer during long-term follow-up, including 6.7 and 11.4 years after their negative evaluations, respectively. We do not have precious answer whether these patients simply have de novo cancer or naturally, genetically potential of malignancy. These data indicate that overwhelming majority of patients who undergo an initial evaluation of urinary tract without any positive findings possibly remain cancer-free. If the urinalysis would be negative for two consecutive years, the risk of urological disease may be no greater than that of the general population [5].

Conclusion

We need to be cautious to distinguish patients with macroscopic hematuria from those with microscopic hematuria. In contrast to the infrequent occurrence of cancer in patients with asymptomatic microscopic hematuria, approximately 25% of those with macroscopic hematuria will be found to have an underlying urinary tract malignancy, and 34% of those are due to the other significant urologic diseases [8, 27].

We think and believe the aim of management of hematuria should be a prompt detection and a treatment of underlying serious causes of hematuria. However, redundant and long-lasting examination and follow-up would not be required. Further studies are warranted the overcoming this classic but important and typical urologic symptom.

References

[1]   Sutton JM: Evaluation of hematuria in adults. *JAMA*. 1990;263:2475-80.

[2]   Woolhandler S, Pels RJ, Bor DH, et al.: Dipstick urinalysis screening of asymptomatic adults for urinary tract disorders. I. Hematuria and proteinuria. *JAMA* 1989;262:1214-19.

[3]   Grossfield GD, Wolf JS, Litwin MS et al.: Asymptomatic microscopic haematuria in adults: summary of the AUA Best Practice Policy Recommendations. *Am. Fam. Physician* 2001;69:870-84.

[4]   Messing EM, Young TB, Hunt VE, et al: Home screening for hematuria: results of a multiclinic study. *J. Urol.* 148:289,1992.

[5]   Davis R, Jones JS, Barocas DA, et al.: Diagnosis, evaluation and follow-up of asymptomatic microhematuria (AMH) in adults: AUA guideline. *J. Urol.* 2012;188:2473-81.

[6]   Schwartz GL: Proper evaluation of asymptomatic microscopic hematuria in the era of evidence-based medicine. Progress is being made. *Mayo Clin.Proceeding.* 2013.88.123-125.

[7]   Cohen RA, Brown RS: Microscopic haematuria. *N. Engl. J. Med.* 2003;348:2330-7.

[8]   Khadra MH, Pickard RS, Charlton M, et al.: A prospective analysis of 1930 patients with hematuria to evaluate current diagnostic practice. *J. Urol.* 2001;163:524-527.

[9]   Carroll PR: Urothelial carcinoma, cancers of bladder, ureter and renal pelvis; In Tanagho EA, McAninch JW eds; Smith's General Urology, 15th edition, Chap21. McGraw-Hill, 355-77.

[10]   Mohr DN, Offord KP, Owen RA, et al.: Asymptomatic microhematuria and urological disease. A population based study. *JAMA*1986;256:224-229.

[11]   Kumar P, Jones JS: How to evaluate 'dipstick hematuria': What to do before you refer. Cleveland clinic. *J. Med.* 2008;75:227-233.

[12]   Matsumoto K, Irie A, Satoh T, et al.: Occupational bladder cancer: from chort study to biologic molecular marker. *Med. Sci. Monit.* 2005;11:RA311-315.

[13]   Britton JP, Dowell AC, Whelan P, et al: A community study of bladder cancer screening by the detection of occult urinary bleeding. *J. Urol,* 1992;148(3):788-90.

[14]   Thompson IM: The evaluation of microscopic hematuria: a population-based study. *J. Urol,* 1987;138(5):1189-90.

[15]   Golin AL, Howard RS: Asymptomatic microscopic hematuria. *J. Urol.*1980;137:527

[16]   Culclasure TF, Bray VJ, Hasbargen JA: The signidicance of hematuria in the anticoagulated patient *Arch. Inter. Med.* 1994;154:649-52.

[17]   Rife CC, Farrow GM, Utz DC: Urine cytology of transitional cell neoplasms. *Urol. Clin North Am.* 1979;6:599.

[18]   Hofland CA, Marani AJ: Is cytology required for a haematuria evaluation. *J. Urol.* 2004;171:324-6.

[19]   Grossfeld GD, Carroll PR: Evaluation of asymptomatic microscopic hematuria. *Urol. Clin. North Am.* 1998;25:661-76.

[20]   Mariani AJ, Mariani MC, Macchioni C, et al.: The significance of adult hematuria: 1000 hematuria evaluations including a risk benefit and cost-effectiveness analysis. *J. Urol.*1989;141:350-5.

[21]   Lang EK, Davis R, Myers L, at al.: Multiphasic Helical Computerized Tomography for the Assessment of Microscopic Hematuria: A Prospective Study. *J. Urol.* 2004;171:237-43.

[22]   Albani JM, Ciashini MW, Streem SB, et al.: The role of computerized tomographic urography in the initial evaluation of hematuria. *J. Urol.* 2007;177:644-8.

[23]   Dunnick NR, Sandler CM, Amis ES Jr, et al.: Functional renal anatomy, renal physiology, and contract media. In: Mitchell CW, ed. Textbook of uroradiology. 2nd ed. Baltimore: Williams & Wilkins, 1997:86-115.

[24]   Miah S, Dudziec E, Drayton RM at al.: An evaluation of urinary microRNA rebveals a high sensitivity for bladder cancer. *Br. J. Cancer.* 2012;107:123-128.

[25]   Kuruma H, Egawa S, Oh-Ishi M, et al.: High molecular mass proteome of androgen-independent prostate cancer. *Proteomics,* 2005.

[26] Madeb R, Golijanin D, Knopf J, et al.: Long-term outcome of patients with a negative work-up for asymptomatic microhematuria. *Urology*. 2010;75:20-5.

[27] Alishahi S, Byrne D, Goodman CM, et al.: Haematuria investigation based on a standard protocol: emphasis on the diagnosis of urological malignancy. *J. R. Coll. Surg. Edinb.* 2002;47:422-427.

In: Hematuria
Editors: Nikhil Vasdev and G. Boustead

ISBN: 978-1-63463-073-3
© 2015 Nova Science Publishers, Inc.

Chapter 9

The Implications of Referral Targets in the Management and Diagnosis of Urological Malignancies in Patients with Haematuria in UK

Vani Agarwal[1], Nikhil Vasdev[1], Todd Kanzara[1], Andrew C. Thorpe[2], Tim Lane[1], James M. Adshead[1] and Gregory Boustead[1]*

[1]Hertfordshire and South Bedfordshire Urological Cancer Centre,
Department of Urology, Lister Hospital, Stevenage, UK
[2]Department of Urology, Freeman Hospital, Newcastle upon Tyne, UK

Introduction

In this book chapter we present the impact of cancer referral targets on the earlier diagnosis and treatment of patients with urological cancers in the United Kingdom (UK). When a patient is seen in primary care in the UK with haematuria, the patients symptoms are assessed and categorized into visible haematuria (VH) versus non-visible haematuria (NVH).

The Renal Association and British Association of Urological Surgeons formed joint guidelines in July 2008 on the initial assessment of patients with haematuria. This was done following a large review that highlighted major deficiencies in the quality assessment of diagnostic criteria [1]. Under current NHS practice, all urology departments have to comply with the '2-week' target for suspected cancer referrals [2]. This target states that all patients with signs or symptoms suggestive of cancer are guaranteed to see a specialist within 2 weeks of their general practitioner requesting an urgent appointment. These guidelines were put in place to allow swift referrals from primary to secondary care teams in the management of patients with suspected cancer.

* Correspondence – nikhilvasdev@doctors.org.uk.

Current Guidelines

NICE have made specific referral guidelines with regards to different urological malignancies [3]. The conditions for urgent referral (within 2 weeks) have been summarized below:

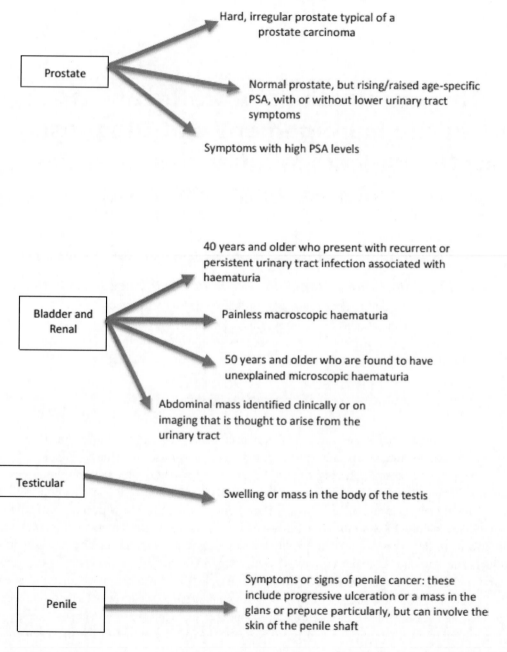

In general, all patients with visible haematuria, symptomatic non-visible haematuria and patients over the age of 40 with asymptomatic non-visible haematuria require direct referral to urology for further investigation. Patients that present with haematuria that do not meet the criteria for referral to urology or nephrology require long term monitoring to assess progression of symptoms and determine the underlying diagnosis.

Gross haematuria is estimated to account for 4% to 20% of all urological hospital visits [4]. The main aim of the '2 week rule' is to allow rapid access for urological patients including patients with painless haematuria, microscopic haematuria, testicular mass, palpable renal mass, raised PSA (prostate-specific antigen) and suspected penile cancer. Earlier stage of presentation is thought to lead to better outcomes- for example Hollenbeck et al. (2010) [5] recently showed that a delay in the diagnosis of bladder cancer increased the risk of death from disease independent of tumour grade and or disease stage. They studied around 30,000 patients with bladder cancer and found that patients who had a diagnosis delay of 9 months were more likely to die from bladder cancer compared with patients who were diagnosed within 3 months with the risk not markedly attenuated after adjusting for disease stage and tumour grade. In that study, the effect was strongest among patients who had low-grade tumours and low-stage disease. This highlights the potential importance of the two-week-wait in improving patient outcomes. However, the effectiveness of the '2 week rule' in the early diagnosis of urological malignancies has to be weighed up with the economic burden of investigating haematuria of patients with no significant pathological condition.

A recent study [6] compared the details of two groups of referrals during the era where there was no '2 week rule' (N= 1,930, April 1994 to March 1997) with the era after the introduction of the '2 week rule' (N=1,740, April 2003 to March 2006). The data showed a 57% increase in the incidence of urological malignancy after the introduction of the '2 week rule'. There was a marked increase in the diagnosis of cancers in the post-introduction of the '2 week rule' group- 86 more new cases of transitional cell carcinoma of the bladder, 16 more new cases of renal cell carcinomas and 28 more cases of prostate cancer. The results of the study ultimately showed an increase in the diagnosis of urological malignancies after the introduction of the two-week-wait, highlighting the benefits of having cancer targets in the NHS.

A study showed that since the introduction of the '2 week rule' the overall time from referral to treatment has reduced by 24% ($P<0.001$) [7]. This suggests that the target has achieved its major aim. However, it has also led to a significant increase in workload for urology departments across the country with a larger number of patients being referred with microscopic haematuria who are unlikely to have significant pathology [8]. In the study, microscopic haematuria made up 16% of all two week wait referrals and no cancer was detected in any of these patients. Another concern is that speeding up referrals may not leave enough time to get all the relevant investigations done before the appointment which could potentially reduce the effectiveness of the appointment. This would be particularly relevant in cases with scrotal disease and haematuria where imaging or urinary cytology tests are often required for diagnosis. A study published in 2008 suggested the need for the refinement of the criteria for the two-week-wait as it found that some of the current guidelines are leading to the referral of patients with a low cancer risk [9].

Since the introduction of the NHS Cancer Plan [10] the impact on waiting times and outcomes has been questionable [11,12]. Specifically with regards to bladder cancer, where the 2-week wait rule relies on the detection of haematuria in order to identify patients with a suspected tumour. Previous studies have reported that the incidence of bladder cancer in patients with microscopic haematuria is less than 5% and these patients may, therefore, be subjected to over-investigation [10] There is no discrepancy between investigating patients with microscopic or macroscopic haematuria; the use of a generic proforma has resulted in a change in focus with macroscopic haematuria patients being investigated through the same pathway. This has had an impact upon the number of urgent referrals.

In conclusion the introduction of urgent cancer targets i.e., the 2 week wait rules in the UK has lead to an increase in the diagnosis of bladder cancer and current literature indicates that the incidence of diagnosing a urological malignancy [6,13] is higher in patients with gross visible haematuria in comparison to non-visible haematuria.

References

[1] Rodgers, M., Nixon, J., Hempel, S., Aho, T., Kelly, J., Neal, D., Duffy, S., Ritchie, G., Kleijnen, J., Westwood, M., 2006. Diagnostic tests and algorithms used in the investigation of haematuria: systematic reviews and economic evaluation. Health Technol Assess 10, iii–iv, xi–259.

[2] Health, D. of, 1999. HSC 1999/205: Cancer waiting times achieving the two week target [WWW Document]. URL http://webarchive.nationalarchives.gov.uk/+/ www.dh.gov.uk/en/Publicationsndstatistics/Lettersandcirculars/Healthservicecirculars/ DH_4004481

[3] NICE: Referral guidelines for suspected cancer [WWW Document], n.d. URL http://www.eguidelines.co.uk/eguidelinesmain/external_guidelines/nice/suspcted_cance r.htm

[4] Mariani, A.J., Mariani, M.C., Macchioni, C., Stams, U.K., Hariharan, A., Moriera, A., 1989. The significance of adult hematuria: 1,000 hematuria evaluations including a risk-benefit and cost-effectiveness analysis. J. Urol. 141, 350–355.

[5] Hollenbeck, B.K., Dunn, R.L., Ye, Z., Hollingsworth, J.M., Skolarus, T.A., Kim, S.P., Montie, J.E., Lee, C.T., Wood, D.P., Jr, Miller, D.C., 2010. Delays in diagnosis and bladder cancer mortality. Cancer 116, 5235–5242.

[6] Vasdev, N., Thorpe, A., 2011. Has the introduction of the "2 week rule" in the UK led to an earlier diagnosis of urological malignancy? Ecancermedicalscience 2011;5:215. doi: 10.3332/ecancer.2011.215.

[7] Blick, C., Bailey, D., Haldar, N., Bdesha, A., Kelleher, J., Muneer, A., 2010. The impact of the two-week wait rule on the diagnosis and management of bladder cancer in a single UK institution. Ann. R. Coll. Surg. Engl. 92, 46–50.

[8] Allen, D., Popert, R., O'Brien, T., 2004. The two-week-wait cancer initiative in urology: useful modernization? J. R. Soc. Med. 97, 279–281.

[9] Hawary, A.M., Warburton, H.E., Brough, R.J., Collins, G.N., Brown, S.C., O'Reilly, P.H., Adeyoju, A.A., 2008. The "2-week wait" rule for referrals for suspected urological cancers--urgent need for refinement of criteria. Ann. R. Coll. Surg. Engl. 90, 517–522.

[10] Department of Health, editor. The NHS Cancer Plan. London: Stationary Office; 2000.

[11] Boman H, Hedelin H, Holmang S. The results of routine evaluation of adult patients with haematuria analysed according to referral form information with 2-year follow-up. Scand. J. Urol. Nephrol.2001;35:497–501.

[12] Hanna SJ, Muneer A, Khalil KH. The 2-week wait for suspected cancer: time for a rethink? *Int. J. Clin. Pract.* 2005;59:1334–9.

[13] Vasdev N, Thorpe A. Should the presence of a culture positive urinary tract infection exclude patients from rapid evaluation hematuria protocols? *Urol. Oncol.* 2013 Aug;31(6):909-13.

In: Hematuria
Editors: Nikhil Vasdev and G. Boustead

ISBN: 978-1-63463-073-3
© 2015 Nova Science Publishers, Inc.

Chapter 10

Hematuria: An American Perspective

Dane E. Klett[1] and Y. Mark Hong[2]
[1]Vattikuti Urology Institute, Henry Ford Health System, Detroit, Michigan, US
[2]Affiliated Urologists, Creighton University School of Medicine, Phoenix, Arizona, US

Introduction

Blood in the urine, known simply as hematuria, is caused by a wide variety of pathologies ranging from benign to life-threatening. It is imperative clinicians understand how to identify hematuria, orchestrate a proper work-up, initiate treatment, and provide adequate follow-up. The prevalence of hematuria ranges from 2.1 to 31.6% depending on the study, and diagnosis and management of the condition is associated with significant healthcare-related costs in the United States [1]. In this chapter we will focus on understanding hematuria in its entirety including the prevalence, causes, diagnosis, management, and expected outcomes of the condition.

Definition

Hematuria is broadly classified as gross or microscopic. Gross hematuria (GH) is defined as urine discoloration due to blood and may occur with the presence of as little as 1 ml of blood per 1 L of urine [2]. Microscopic hematuria (MH) is defined by the American Urological Association (AUA) as the presence of three or more red blood cells (RBCs) per high-power field (HPF), in the absence of infection or contamination, in one properly collected urine sample [1]. It is important to note that while previous MH definitions required 2-3 positive urine samples, the most recent 2012 AUA Guideline on hematuria requires only a single positive urine sample to initiate a work-up [1]. The definition was updated to account for the highly intermittent nature of hematuria and the theoretical possibility of missing serious pathology, including malignancy, as well as the potential for the MH work-up to uncover non-life threatening conditions for which active management could provide patient benefit.

Epidemiology

The incidence of hematuria varies widely among the general population. Multiple factors including age, gender, smoking habit, exposure history, geographic location, screening frequency, and hematuria definition have led to a wide variability in study data. According to data compiled by the AUA from multiple published studies representing over 80,000 patients, rates of hematuria range from 2.4% to 31.1% among the general population [1]. Higher rates are seen in males, those greater than age 60, those with smoking history, and those with a higher screening frequency [1]. Higher hematuria rates among these individuals are directly related to the increased incidence of urologic disease seen in this demographic. Though published data on the prevalence of hematuria varies widely among the general population health-care providers should expect to see patients suffering from hematuria due to the wide variety of associated pathologies, and understand the need for further investigation.

Etiology

Hematuria is associated with several conditions. In this section we will discuss the more common conditions associated with gross and/or microscopic hematuria.

Traditionally, hematuria is separated into categories, glomerular or extra-glomerular, based on the anatomic site from which the bleeding originates. Glomerular hematuria is associated with the presence of RBC casts, dysmorphic RBCs, and/or proteinuria. The most common causes of glomerular hematuria include nephropathies, such as membranous nephropathy, or nephritis, such as IgA nephritis, which are commonly immunological, infectious or drug-induced in nature [1]. If a glomerular source of bleeding is identified, especially in the presence of proteinuria, it is best to involve an experienced nephrologist in the care of the patient to ensure proper medical management of the kidney.

Extra-glomerular hematuria refers to any bleeding source found outside of the glomeruli. It is often associated with normal appearing RBCs and blood clots, but lacks evidence of RBC casts or proteinuria. Extra-glomerular hematuria may originate from many locations within the genitourinary (GU) tract including the kidneys, ureters, bladder, prostate, and urethra. Generally, the differential for extra-glomerular hematuria is broad and etiologies include: vascular conditions (malformations and infarcts), infections, inflammation, trauma, post-surgical, exercise-induced, autoimmune disease, metabolic conditions (calculi), medications (cyclophosphamide), and neoplasms (benign and malignant).

It is also important to keep in mind red-colored urine does not always equate to a urinary bleeding source. Physicians should consider all possible sources of bleeding. For example, a woman presenting on her menstrual period with hematuria may represent urine contamination rather than primary urinary bleeding. Red-colored urine also does not always signify hematuria. In fact, many other substances can lead to red-colored urine. Examples include pigment from the body (myoglobin), pigment from foods (beets), and pigment from medications (phenazopyridine) to name a few.

Overall, infection accounts for about 25% of all hematuria cases [5]. Calculi are the second leading cause, accounting for approximately 20% of hematuria cases [6]. In about 10% of cases, no cause or source of bleeding is ever discovered, an entity termed benign, idiopathic hematuria [7]. Anti-coagulants may trigger hematuria, particularly in patients with pre-existing bleeding sources such as bladder cancer or an enlarged prostate. However, these patients should still receive a thorough work-up after gross hematuria has been stabilized.

Diagnosis

The first step in the hematuria work-up, as with any entity in medicine, is a thorough history and directed physical exam. History should include a discussion of the current symptoms including onset, severity, frequency, and timing, taking care to address related symptoms such as fever, pain, irritative voiding symptoms, rash, and joint complaints. It is also important to inquire about recent diet, illness, exercise, surgeries, and/or trauma. Also pertinent are the social history (tobacco use, environmental or chemical exposures, and work history), medical history (medications, urologic disease, and radiation exposure), surgical history, and family history (hematuria and urologic malignancies). After gathering sufficient history a directed physical exam is performed.

The physical exam should begin with exam of the skin for any signs of rash or infection. The back and abdomen should be palpated to assess for tenderness or the presence of an abdominal mass such as renal mass or palpable bladder. Lastly, in both males and females, the external genitalia should be thoroughly examined for lesions. In males a prostate exam, and in females a targeted pelvic exam, should be performed.

The second step in the work-up for hematuria is a urinalysis, which includes the urine dipstick and microscopy. The urine sample should be a clean-catch, mid-stream sample with few squamous cells. If mid-stream collection is unobtainable the physician may consider obtaining a catheterized sample directly from the bladder. The urine dipstick test is often done first, and is designed to assess for the presence of hemoglobin. Hemoglobin is structurally similar to other compounds including myoglobin (found in muscle) and certain bacterial peroxidases, which may lead to false-positive results [2]. False-negative results may be seen with vitamin C ingestion, urine pH of less than 5.1, and with a dipstick that has been subject to prolonged air exposure prior to testing [3,4]. Regardless, if the urine dipstick is positive, or high suspicion of hematuria remains in light of a negative dipstick, urine microscopy is warranted.

Microscopy is used to confirm the presence of and characterize RBCs (normal or dysmorphic), and to look for casts or proteinuria. According to the 2012 AUA guidelines, a diagnosis of hematuria is confirmed with three or greater RBCs per HPF in a single urine sample [1]. If elements other than normal RBCs are present, such as dysmorphic RBCs, proteinuria or cellular casts, patients should undergo a nephrology evaluation in addition to the continued assessment of a urologic cause [1]. If hematuria has been caused by a benign condition, such as infection, it should be properly treated and the urinalysis repeated at a later date. If the urinalysis is negative at follow-up no further work-up is necessary. If benign causes of hematuria have been excluded, and/or hematuria continues despite previous treatment, then further urologic work-up is warranted [1].

If further hematuria work-up is being considered it is important to obtain a baseline set of laboratory values. Physicians should obtain a blood urea nitrogen (BUN), creatinine, and estimated glomerular filtration rate (eGFR) to assess kidney function. These labs are important to review before considering imaging modalities or procedural anesthesia, especially if intravenous contrast administration is planned. Physicians may also want to consider obtaining a complete blood count to assess for anemia or an elevated white blood cell count that may need to be addressed.

The next step in the urologic work-up of hematuria is radiologic imaging and cystoscopy. The best imaging modality in the work-up for hematuria is the computed tomography urogram (CTU). It allows for proper evaluation of both the renal parenchyma and upper tracts. According to AUA guidelines 2012, in patients with adequate renal function, a CTU with and without contrast should be obtained and include an excretory phase to evaluate the collecting system bilaterally [1]. If CTU is contraindicated magnetic resonance urography (MRU) with and without contrast is an acceptable alternative and retrograde pyelograms (RPGs) may be obtained if adequate imaging of the upper tracts is required [1]. Lastly, in patients with contraindications to CTU with contrast and MRU such as patients with impaired renal function, physicians may consider obtaining a non-contrast CT, renal ultrasound (US) or RPGs [1].

Cystoscopy is utilized to assess the condition of the urethra, bladder, and ureteral orifices. It is a relatively simple procedure that may be done in the office setting under local anesthesia or operating room under IV sedation or general anesthesia depending on the needs of the patient. According to 2012 AUA guidelines, cystoscopy, without the use of blue light, is recommended for all patients 35 years of age and older or for any patient at an increased risk for urologic malignancy including: patients with irritative voiding symptoms, history of tobacco use, history of radiation, and/or history of chemical carcinogen exposure [1]. It is best performed following review of radiologic imaging. This allows physicians to inspect, in real-time, any lesions found on imaging. It also enables physicians, if necessary, to perform ureteroscopy, tissue biopsies, clot evacuation, further imaging studies, and/or other assessments in a single procedure. Of note, although blue light cystoscopy has been shown in limited studies to have a higher sensitivity versus standard cystoscopy the standard of care in America does not warrant its use at this time [8]. Further evidence regarding outcomes and cost effectiveness are necessary before implementation of blue light cystoscopy.

Of final note is the use of cytology and urine tumor markers such as NMP22, BTA-stat, and UroVysion FISH in the work-up of hematuria. According to 2012 AUA guidelines, use of cytology and/or urine markers is not indicated in the routine work-up of hematuria due to the high degree of unreliability associated with the tests [1]. Cytology, however, may be warranted in patients who continue to experience hematuria despite a negative work-up or patients with serious carcinoma-related risk factors such as irritative voiding symptoms, history of tobacco use, and/or chemical exposure [1]. It is also unclear whether urine markers may one day be able to replace cystoscopy as the diagnostic test of choice in terms of accuracy and cost-effectiveness [9].

Management

The management of hematuria varies and is cause-dependent. Treatment of glomerular disease should involve a nephrologist. In cases of extra-glomerular bleeding, urologists and physicians dealing with GU conditions should follow appropriate treatment guidelines. Treatment of primary causes, for example hematuria secondary to renal cell carcinoma, would proceed if the hematuria is not severe enough to be acutely symptomatic, anemic or cause hemodynamic instability. In cases of moderate to severe gross hematuria, with or without the presence of blood clots, acute management of bleeding may be necessary to prevent life-threating complications. The remainder of this section will focus specifically on the acute management of gross hematuria.

Gross hematuria may be observed in a variety of locations including the office setting, emergency room, and wards. It is imperative physicians understand how to manage this condition as well as associated complications including obstructive renal failure, anemia and even bladder perforation. As a general rule patients on anti-coagulants, such as warfarin or heparin, and non-steroidal anti-inflammatories, such as ibuprofen or aspirin, should discontinue these medications immediately. Such decisions should always be coordinated with the patient's care primary care and cardiology team.

The key concept, and one of the least understood aspects of hematuria management in the hospital, is to first remove clots from the bladder. Gross hematuria will not clear without first removing existing clots from the bladder, which likely has to do with the action of urokinase in urine (further discussion below). This is generally accomplished by placement of a large bore Foley catheter. Standard Foley catheters in the United States are 16 French, which is usually of inadequate radial size to allow proper flow and therefore irrigation of clots. Poiseuille's Law governs this interaction in that flow rate through a tube is affected by radius of the tube to the fourth power. A standard 16 French Foley has a diameter of 5.3 mm, or radius of 2.7 mm. A 22 French Foley has a diameter of 7.3 mm, or radius of 3.7 mm. Even though the radius of a 22 French Foley is only 1 mm more than a 16 French Foley, there is 3.6 times more flow through a 22 French Foley than a 16 French Foley based on Poiseuille's Law.

Therefore, a 20 or 22 French two-way catheter should be requested immediately for severe cases of gross hematuria. This process often takes time to deliver to the patient bedside because a 22 French Foley is not a standard piece of equipment stocked in American emergency rooms or hospital floors. Another key distinction is to start by irrigating the large-bore Foley manually, not with a 3-way Foley. A 3-way Foley is also often misleadingly labeled as a "hematuria" catheter. It contains an extra port and channel for irrigant to run into the bladder and the usual channel that allows urine to drain out. Due to the need to fit an extra irrigation channel into a Foley, the outflow channel is much smaller in a 3-way Foley versus a 2-way Foley of the same French size (again, consider Poiseuille's Law). Since the key concept is to first evacuate existing blood clots from the bladder, a manually-irrigated large bore 2-way Foley will accomplish this goal better than with a same-sized large bore 3-way Foley.

Another mistake often made in emergency rooms, ICU's and hospital floors is the "knee-jerk" reaction of initially placing a 3-way Foley for gross hematuria and starting continuous bladder irrigation (CBI). CBI is a process whereby a bag of irrigant, usually normal saline, is put on an IV pole at higher elevation relative to the patient and connected to tubing that allows irrigant to flow into the inflow channel of a 3-way Foley. Doing so often gives a false sense of security in the acute setting because the inflow irrigant may temporarily "clear up" gross hematuria in the outflow channel. However, if blood clots have not been first manually evacuated out, then there is the risk of worsening the situation by running in more fluid via CBI into a bladder that is already full of clots. This can lead to inadvertent bladder rupture, especially if CBI is connected to an IV pump for continuous flow, which should *never* be done. Therefore, the initial management of gross hematuria with clots is to place a large-bore, 2-way Foley and manually irrigate with normal saline and a catheter tip 60 cc syringe. This process is laborious and time-consuming at times. If after a long period of time, clots are continuing to be drawn back in the syringe or there is a sense that clots are not being evacuated despite manual irrigation, decision may be made for cystoscopy and evacuation of clots in the operating room.

Once clots have been completely evacuated from the bladder, then a large bore (20 or 22 French) 3-way Foley can be placed and CBI started. The concept here is that once the bladder is free of clots, CBI will then help prevent new clots from forming. In the meantime, other sources of bleeding such as supratherapeutic anticoagulation can be addressed. CBI can be gradually decreased by nursing staff and manual irrigation can be intermittently performed every 1-4 hours depending on the severity of hematuria to make sure no new clots have formed that require evacuation while on CBI. Once hematuria remains stable or clear off CBI, then the irrigation channel port can be plugged and CBI stopped. Keep in mind, after acute symptomatic gross hematuria has been stabilized, an investigation to determine the cause of hematuria is always indicated, especially to rule out occult malignancy.

Special situations include the management of post-prostate procedure hematuria such as transurethral resection of the prostate (TURP). Traction may be placed on the catheter in an effort to tamponade bleeding. Traction is best achieved by placing a catheter in the bladder, filling the balloon with sterile water (at times filling the balloon up to 30 cc or more depending on the size of prostate resection), tying a surgical sponge to the external portion of the catheter proximal to the drainage ports, gently applying traction to the catheter while simultaneously sliding the surgical sponge to the tip of the penis, and securing the external portion of the catheter to the mid-thigh with the use of either foam tape or a pre-manufactured leg strap. In general, traction should be used carefully to avoid prolonged periods of traction time and decrease risk of penile devascularization.

Despite previous efforts, hematuria may continue and other, more definitive, treatment may be required. Cystoscopy and CT urogram or retrograde pyelogram in the operative room may identify bleeding etiology. There are three main anatomic sites of concern for gross hematuria: bladder, prostate, and kidneys.

Gross hematuria originating in the bladder is most often associated with infection, medication, and/or malignancy. Management of persistent hematuria includes CBI, use of anti-bleeding agents in conjunction with CBI, allowing time for bleeding to cease on its own, and cystoscopy with fulguration and possible instilled medical agents in the operating room. First is the use of aminocaproic acid, a plasmin inhibitor, to decrease the breakdown of clots and encourage hemostasis. It is delivered three ways. The intravenous (IV) route is dosed at 5 g of aminocaproic acid per 250 mL of normal saline which is infused over one hour. This is followed by 1 gram per hour IV infusion over the next eight hours or until bleeding is resolved. The oral route is given as an initial 5 g oral dose followed by a 1 g oral dose every hour. The final, and possibly safest route, is intravesical instillation with CBI at a dose of 1 g of aminocaproic acid per 1 liter of normal saline. Contraindications to this treatment include disseminated intravascular coagulation, upper tract, or patients at risk for thrombosis. A serious complication of this treatment is rhabdomyolysis which should be monitored via creatinine phosphokinase (CPK) levels in patients undergoing this treatment for greater than 24 hours.

Another treatment option involves the instillation of intravesical hemostatic agents including alum, silver nitrate, and formalin. Of the three, alum is the only agent that may be instilled without the use of general anesthesia, may be given to patients with vesicoureteral reflux (VUR), and is not known to cause scarring of the bladder. Alum is prepared by mixing 10 g of aluminum potassium sulfate, or aluminum ammonium sulfate, with 1 liter of distilled water. Once blood clots are evacuated from the bladder the 1% alum solution may be instilled at a maximum rate of 300 ml per hour. Bleeding usually resolves within 72 to 96 hours. Complications of this treatment include systemic alum absorption which is associated with increased levels of aluminum, potassium, and/or ammonia, depending on the mixture chosen. These levels should be monitored in all patients, especially those with renal insufficiency as it may accumulate systemically. If symptoms develop, such as palpitations or changes in mentation, alum instillation should be discontinued.

Another intravesical agent that may be used is silver nitrate. This causes pain and should be done under spinal or general anesthesia. A cystogram is required prior to instillation to rule out VUR and extravasation. If VUR is present, Fogarty catheters may be placed to occlude the ureteral orifices, and a repeat cystogram should be done to ensure no reflux is present. All clots must be evacuated from the bladder prior to instillation. Silver nitrate 0.5% to 1% mixed with sterile water is used. An 18F Foley catheter is placed into the bladder and light traction is applied to prevent silver nitrate from entering the urethra. The silver nitrate solution is then instilled into the bladder under gravity and the catheter is clamped for 10 to 20 minutes. After the appropriate time has passed, the clamp is removed, the silver nitrate solution is drained, and the bladder irrigated with normal saline. Bleeding normally resolves in 24 to 48 hours using this agent. Complications associated with this treatment are related to its caustic nature, and severe scarring is possible.

The final intravesical agent is formalin. It is the most effective intravesical agent, but the most caustic and painful, and should be reserved for the most severe cases. It requires instillation under spinal or general anesthesia. A cystogram is required prior to instillation to rule out VUR and extravasation. If VUR is present, Fogarty catheters may be placed to occlude the ureteral orifices, and a repeat cystogram should be done to ensure no reflux is present. The perineum should be coated with a layer of petroleum jelly, and in females the vagina should be packed with petroleum jelly gauze. This is done to limit the caustic effects of formalin on bare skin and mucosa. All clots must be evacuated from the bladder prior to instillation. Formalin 4% in distilled water is used. An 18F Foley catheter is placed into the bladder and light traction is applied to prevent the formalin solution from entering the urethra. The formalin solution is then instilled into the bladder under gravity and the catheter is clamped for 10 minutes. After the appropriate time has passed, the clamp is removed, the formalin solution is drained, and the bladder irrigated with normal saline. Bleeding normally resolves in 48 hours. This process may be repeated using concentrations of formalin up to 10%. Complications associated with this treatment are also related to its caustic nature, and severe scarring can ensue.

Physicians may consider surgical treatment options for the management of refractory gross hematuria. One option is to place nephrostomy tubes, which are tubes placed directly into the kidneys that divert urine from the bladder. Urine, which contains the plasmin activating enzyme urokinase, can inhibit hemostasis. Without urokinase in the bladder to activate the clot lysis cascade, hemostasis may be achieved. Another option is embolization or ligation of the bladder. This option targets the bladder's blood supply, the internal iliac artery, and can be effective though not without risks such as devascularizing other structures. Both embolization and nephrostomy tubes are generally placed by Interventional Radiologists in the United States. Lastly, a cystectomy may be considered for life-saving circumstances or in cases where all other options have been ineffective.

Gross hematuria originating in the prostate is most often associated with recent instrumentation, benign prostatic hyperplasia (BPH), infection, and/or malignancy. Multiple therapies are utilized in refractory cases. Aminocaproic acid is a reasonable option and proper administration guidelines are discussed above. Cystoscopic procedures, such as electrocautery fulguration with roller ball or TURP, are also options to control bleeding. Lastly, an open prostatectomy may be considered in life-threatening circumstances or in cases where all other less invasive options have been ineffective.

Gross hematuria originating in the kidneys is most often associated with trauma, infection, calculi, renal disease, recent surgery, and/or malignancy. Managing refractory cases can be difficult. Systemic administration of hemostatic agents such as aminocaproic acid or alum can be considered, one must consider the benefits versus te risk of ureteral obstruction from clots. Embolization of the main renal artery, or the specific branch associated with bleeding source, can be considered in serious cases and if unsuccessful, partial or total nephrectomy can be considered.

After the patient is stabilized and adequate hemostasis is achieved, a proper hematuria work-up should be performed. This is especially important following episodes of gross hematuria because urologic malignancy is found in up to 23% of patients as compared to 5% with microscopic hematuria [10].

Follow-Up

If an etiology is established during the initial hematuria work-up, patients should undergo proper treatment for their respective disease and follow-up accordingly. If the initial hematuria work-up is negative, follow-up remains important. In 43% of microscopic hematuria patients and 8% of gross hematuria patients, initial work-up fails to identify an etiology [10]. Despite a negative initial work-up approximately 3% of microscopic hematuria patients, and 18% of gross hematuria patients, go on to develop a urologic malignancy [10]. According to 2012 AUA guidelines, patients with a negative initial work-up following an episode of microscopic hematuria should receive annual urinalyses [1]. After two consecutive negative annual urinalyses, patients may be released from care [1]. If hematuria persists urinalyses should be done yearly and a full work-up should be repeated at three to five years [1]. In patients with gross hematuria no official guideline recommendations exist, although in the presence of risk factors such as smoking history, one can consider an earlier follow-up schedule. Lastly, it is important to instruct all patients, especially those with significant risk factors for GU malignancy, that if the hematuria worsens or returns they should return for evaluation as serious underlying pathology may be present.

Special Situations

Hematuria in pregnant females is a situation that requires special consideration. Although the majority of cases are benign, up to 5% are associated with GU malignancy [1]. Also, common, benign causes of hematuria such as infection may result in fetal complications if not properly identified and treated. Following urinalysis, the 2012 AUA Guidelines recommend pregnant females be screened for major renal lesions using MRU, MRI with RPGs, or US during pregnancy, and a full work-up should be done after delivery [1].

Conclusion

Hematuria is a common condition and is caused by a variety of pathologies ranging from benign to life-threatening. Physicians must understand how to properly identify hematuria and stratify risk with history-taking and laboratory data. Proper radiologic imaging and endoscopic procedures must be performed to determine the etiology of the hematuria and proper treatment initiated of the hematuria to stabilize patients in the short-term and treat the primary etiology in the long-term. Adequate follow-up ensures patients at greatest risk for GU malignancy and non-malignant disease are properly screened over time.

References

[1]   Davis R, Jones JS, Barocas DA, et al. Diagnosis, evaluation, and follow-up of asymptomatic microhematuria (AMH) in adults: AUA Guideline. *American Urological Association (AUA) Guideline* 2012.

[2]   Fatica R, Fowler A. Hematuria. *Cleveland Clinic: Current Clinical Medicine* 2nd Edi. Carey WD, Nurko S. Philadelphia, Saunders, Ch. 9, 845-848.

[3]   Grossfeld GD, Carroll PR. Evaluation of asymptomatic microscopic hematuria. *Urol. Clin. North Am.* 1998;25(4):661-6.

[4]   Thaller TR, Wang LP. Evaluation of asymptomatic microscopic hematuria in adults. *Am. Fam. Physician 1999;*60(4):1143-52.

[5]   Heller JE. Asymptomatic microhematuria and urologic disease. A population-based study. *JAMA* 1986;256(19):224-9.

[6]   Ahmed Z, Lee J. Asymptomatic urinary abnormalities. Hematuria and proteinuria. *Med. Clin. North Am.* 1997;81(3):641-52.

[7]   Sokolosky MC. Hematuria. *Emerg. Med. Clin. North Am.* 2001; 19(3):621-32.

[8]   Lee JS, Lee SY, Kim WJ, et al. Efficacy and safety of hexaminolevulinate fluorescence cystoscopy in the diagnosis of bladder cancer. *Korean J. Urol.* 2012;53(12):821-5.

[9]   Hong YM, Loughlin KR. Economic impact of tumor markers in bladder cancer surveillance. *Urology* 2008;71(1):131-5.

[10] Sutton JM. Evaluation of hematuria in adults. *JAMA* 1990;263(18):2475-80.

In: Hematuria
Editors: Nikhil Vasdev and G. Boustead

ISBN: 978-1-63463-073-3
© 2015 Nova Science Publishers, Inc.

Chapter 11

Hematuria in Children: Etiology, Clinical Implications and Management

J. A. March-Villalba[*]*, I. Povo Martín, A. Polo Rodrigo,*
A. Serrano Durbá and C. Domínguez Hinarejos
Pediatric Urology Unit, Department of Urology,
Hospital Universitario y Politécnico La Fe Valencia España

Introduction

Hematuria can be defined as the presence of red blood cells in urine. It is classified as macroscopic/gross hematuria when urine blood-stained is even with the presence of clots, versus microscopic hematuria where red blood cells are observed using a microscope. The American Urological Association (AUA) recommends a definition for microscopic hematuria as three or more red blood cells per high-power microscopic field in urinary sediment from two of three properly collected urinalysis specimens [1].

The major causes of hematuria differ between children and adults. Painless hematuria in adults is usually related to malignant processes, while hematuria in children is related to a wide spectrum of causes mostly not related to malignancy [2-4].

Asymptomatic gross or microscopic hematuria is relatively common in children. In more than a half of the cases this is due to an easily identifiable cause. [5]

Another important aspect to consider is the accompanying symptoms. Symptomatic hematuria in children is due to urinary tract infection or several conditions depending on the signs and symptoms also associated [4, 6].

In this chapter we provide a description of the different causes of hematuria in childhood (table 1).

---

[*] Corresponding author: Avenida del Maestro Rodrigo 88-37 46015 Valencia España. Phone: +34648131545. Email: joseantoniomarch@hotmail.com.

Table 1. Hematuria causes in childhood

Hematuria causes in childhood related at this chapter

Congenital anomalies
   -Vesicoureteral reflux
   -Ureteropelvic junction obstruction
   -Nutcracker syndrome

Infectious or inflammatory etiology
   -Bacterial cystitis-E. Coli
   -Viral cystitis- Adenovirus type 11
       -Stem cell Transplantation- Polyoma BK

Genitourinary neoplasms
   -Wilms´tumor (nephroblastoma)
   - Rhabdomyosarcoma
   -Transitional cell carcinoma
   -Bladder hemangioma
   -Pheochromocytomas/paragangliomas

Urinary Stone disease

Trauma

Systemic or autoinmune disorders. Nephropathy
   -Acute poststreptococcal glomerulonephritis
   -Hemolytic-uremic syndrome
   -Alport síndrome
   -Familial IgA disease
   -Benign familial hematuria (thin basement membrane nephropathy)
   - Autosomal dominant / recessive polycystic kidney disease
   -Systemic lupus erythematosus
   -Henoch Schoenlein purpura
   -Hereditary hemorrhagic telangiectasia (Osler-Weber-Rendu disease)

Haematological disorders
   -Sickle cell anemia
   -Von Willebrand disease

Induced by drugs or substancies

1.1. Congenital Anomalies

Hematuria as a primary sign of urinary tract anomaly is extremely rare but there are different urological congenital disorders that can produce it. Greenfield et al. found a 13% of congenital anomalies in a child population with gross hematuria. The most frequent associated anomaly was *vesicoureteral reflux*. The majority of patients with concurrent vesicoureteral reflux and gross hematuria had sterile culture results and the most frequent grade of reflux was II-III [2].

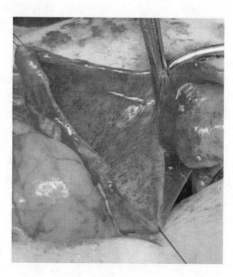

Figure 1. Surgical detail of a renal pelvis urothelial mucosa with vascular congestive areas, in ureteropelvic junction obstruction that may cause hematuria as a result of vascular rupture as pressure increased.

Obstructive lesions, such as *ureteropelvic junction obstruction* may appear with urinary stones and hematuria (figure 1). This situation can be found also in a horseshoe kidney. [7].

The cause of hematuria in a low-grade reflux without infection is unexplained, and the reflux may have been coincidental and an unrelated finding [2].

Another entity that may present with hematuria is the *nutcracker syndrome*. It consists in a mesoaortic compression (between the aorta and the superior mesenteric artery) of the left renal vein. This compression causes venous hypertension, which results in the formation of extra and intrarenal venous collaterals, and subsequent rupture of the septum between the veins and the collecting system, manifesting as intermitent macro/micro hematuria, hypertension and left flank pain. The development of gonadal vein reflux,that may generate pelvic congestion due to pelvic varices does not occur in children [8,9].

First diagnostic procedures ininclude a renal Doppler ultrasound followed by an MRI. Treatment varies from follow-up, placing a ureteral stent in a permanent renoureteral crisis or renocaval reimplantation in less common severe cases [9].

1.2. Infectious or Inflammatory Etiology

Urinary tract infection may cause hematuria. Symptoms vary according to the age of the child. Dysuria, urgency and frequency, usually appear in adolescent and scholar patients. Infants may have general symptoms such as a fever, irritability or apathy, decreased appetite and vomiting. [4]

Etiology may be bacterial or viral. *Bacterial hemorrhagic cystitis* in the abscense of congenital anomalies can occur. Escherichia coli appears to be a much more common cause of acute hemorrhagic cistitis [10]. Hemorragic bacterial cystitis is more common in boys than in girls, unlike to what happens in adult population. It is unclear why this gender predilection exists. High grade vesicoureteral reflux may be related in these situations [2]. The treatment consists an antibiotic prescription and general maneuvers such as fluid intake and painkillers.

Hemorrhagic cystitis due to *viral causes* may be caused in healthy children or in a state of immunosuppresion or immunodepression. The most common cause of viral hemorrhagic cystitis is adenovirus type 11 infections [11]. This viral cystitis is often reported as a cystitis with lack of known etiology because no viral cultures were routinely obtained due to their good prognosis at dismissal [2].

Virus-associated hemorrhagic cystitis is a major cause of morbidity and mortality following allogeneic hematopoietic stem cell transplantation. Hemorrhagic cystitis incidence in recent retrospective studies of pediatric bone-marrow transplant populations still approaches 10-20% [12]. Polyoma BK virus is a more significant cause of hemorrhagic cystitis than adenovirus in children undergoing stem cell transplantation [12,13]. Immune deficiency is more likely to be associated with adenovirus infection, whereas immune hyperactivity might play a key role in polyoma BK virus hemorrhagic cystitis. [14]

Cystoscopy may reveal circumscript papulous tumors as the source of hematuria. Severe and persistent hematuria may require blood transfusions, insertion of large suprapubic catheters and permanent bladder irrigation because of recurrent blood clot retention. Attempts to stop the hematuria coagulation maneuvers may fail to stop the bleeding. In these severe cases, intravesical administration of hyaluronic acid or sodium hyaluronate seems to be effective and safe and may be a promising treatment in patients suffering from severe and late onset hematuria [15-17].

1.3. Genitourinary Neoplasms

Wilms´tumor (nephroblastoma) is the most common intrarenal malignancy of childhood. Wilms' tumor occurs with increased frequency in patients with aniridia, hemihypertrophy, cryptorchidism, hypospadias and other genitourinary abnormalities. The risk of Wilms' tumor is markedly increased in children with Beckwith-Wiedemann syndrome, Drash syndrome, Bloom syndrome and WAGR syndrome (*W*ilms' tumor, *a*niridia, *g*enitourinary malformation and mental *r*etardation). The classic signs and symptoms include abdominal pain, abdominal mass and hematuria. Diagnosis is made according to ultrasound and MRI /CT examinations (figure 2). Treatment is based on the combined approach of chemotherapy, surgery and radiation therapy in advanced cases. [4,18] In this cases hematuria may be may be aggravated by the presence of a coagulopathy (adquired von Willebrand síndrome). [19]

Genitourinary rhabdomyosarcoma is the third most common malignant tumor in children following Wilms´tumor and neuroblastoma. Symptoms and signs include urinary incontinence, urinary tract infections, disuria, urinary retention and hematuria in 25% of the cases [4,20]. Physical examination in boys may reveal a hard-consistency mass in the prostate area, while in females, urethral or vaginal lesions may protude beyond the introitus or the uretral meatus. This tumor can also be found in bladder and differential diagnosis must be made with neuroblastoma and pseudotumor caused by benign cystitis [4,20-22].

Staging of rhabdomyosarcoma is done with CT or MRI. Biopsy should be taken. Treatment is based on chemotheraphy and surgery like radical cystoprostatectomy or partial cystectomy and adjuvant high dose rate brachytherapy [23]. Rabdomyosarcoma survival prognosis is poor [20-23].

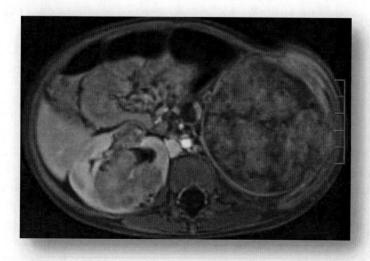

Figure 2. MRI image of bilateral Wilms´tumor (nephroblastoma) that comprises and infiltrates urinary tract.

Transitional cell carcinoma is a very rare malignant neoplasm in children which rarely seen before the age of adolescence. Almost all of these tumors manifest with the presence of hematuria. Diagnosis of transitional cell carcinoma in children is identical to adults. Cystoscopy and transuretral resection must be performed and also a MRI to rule out the existence of tumors in the upper urinary tract [4, 24]. Most of these tumors in young patients are superficial and well differenciated but there is a high recurrence rate [24]. A single dose of mitomycin C instillation after resection was reported to improve recurrence-free survival [25]. Urothelial carcinoma could also appear as a secondary malignancy following chemoteraphy, concrectly cyclophosphamide [4].

Other bladder tumors are for example adenocarcinoma associated to bladder extrophy, but these tumors usually appear after childhood. *Bladder hemangioma* is a benign lesion composed of aberrant blood vessels. Painless hematuria may occur. Diagnosis can be made by Doppler ultrasound revealing a hypervascular tumor in the bladder wall. Cystoscopy may provide the final diagnosis. Special care must be take prior to resection and coagulation, preferably using laser energy [26,27].

Pheochromocytomas/paragangliomas are components of several hereditary cancer syndromes. Up to 30% may be associated with germ-line mutations of genes, including VHL, RET, and SDH. Bladder is a location for these tumors. Final diagnosis is usually established by the histological examination because the macroscopic lesion may a bladder hemangioma or transitional tumor. Partial cystectomy is the treatment option for recurrence [28].

1.4. Urinary Stone Disease

The incidence of urinary tract stone disease has increased significantly in developed countries and it seems that this is due to lifestyle, dietary habits and overweight [29-31]. During childhood it occurs equally, and although the prevalence is lower than in adults, over 1% of all stones occur in patients under 18 years. Urolithiasis in chilhood is a major health problem due to the fact that children are a high risk group for recurrence and the threat of deterioration of renal function and therefore, should be studied for prevention [29-32].

Having a family history of urolithiasis is present in up to half of patients. Risk factors for developing stones are metabolic disorders, infections, urinary tract abnormalities, family history, bladder dysfunction, hypertension and diabetes mellitus in children under 6 years, systemic diseases like renal tubular acidosis, malabsorptive diseases like cystic fibrosis, inflammatory bowel diseases and environmental and dietary factors [29,30, 32-34].

Congenital abnormalities of the urinary tract in association with urolithiasis are about 20%, reaching 79.5% in less than one year old. The most common anomaly is the pyeloureteral stenosis followed by vesicoureteral reflux and neurogenic bladder disease [29,30].

Clinical presentation of urolithiasis in children depends on age, the most common symptoms in older children are flank pain and hematuria, whereas younger children present less specific symptoms with a higher frequency of hematuria, urinary infections and flank pain [33-35].

Microscopic hematuria may be the only indicator of Stone disease and more common in children [33]. However, the absence of hematuria in a patient with flank pain does not exclude the presence of stones, on the other hand, the presence of hematuria and flank pain does not have enough positive predictive value for the diagnosis of urolithiasis [36,37]. A study performed by Moghtaderi et al. screened for microhaematuria on 3,000 children between 6 and 14 years observing its existence in 1.2%, of these, 50% had stones [38].

In patients with stones and gross hematuria percentage reported in the literature varies between 15-30% [31, 39, 40].

Metabolic disorders in patients with stones are present in more than 50% but this percentage varies depending on factors such as age (more common in children), geographic area and sex [34, 35, 39-43]. The most common disorders are hypercalciuria, hyperuricosuria, hyperoxaluria, cystinuria, hypocitraturia and hypomagnesuria. The composition of the most common stones is calcium oxalate to 60% followed by uric acid, calcium phosphate, struvite and cystine [40, 42, 43].

In addition to metabolic evaluation, imaging of the urinary tract such as ultrasound, plain abdominal film, and intravenous urography are suitable diagnostic imaging modalities. Treatment of urinary stones in children is the same as in adults. Children have better chances than adults for spontaneous stone expulsion. Moreover, studies report higher success rates in children with shock wave lithotripsy (SWL), even in large stones. During SWL treatment, a protective lung shield should be applied to prevent shock wave lung contusions. Under these conditions, SWL in children is safe and highly effective [4, 42].

1.5. Trauma

Trauma is the main cause of morbidity and mortality in children. About 3% of children admitted at pediatric hospital trauma centres will have significant genitourinary injuries. These injuries are seldom life-threatening but a thorough history of the events and physical examination must be carried out in order to determine the appropriate urological management of these children [43, 44].

Urological trauma can be caused either by penetrating or, more common by blunt injuries such as falls, motor vehicle accidents, sports injuries, physical assault or sexual abuse. Hematuria is a sign that can be found in children with urinary tract trauma and must be carefully assessed [43, 44].

Kidney is the most frequent site of genitourinary (GU) trauma and up to 80-90% of kidney injuries are due to blunt trauma. The pediatric kidney is more vulnerable to blunt trauma than the adult´s kidney because it is larger in proportion to the body cavity, it has a lower position (the posterior ribs do not protect it as much as they do in adults), abdominal and trunk muscles are less developed and there is less retroperitoneal and perirenal fat [43-45].

Kidneys with congenital abnormalities are more vulnerable to blunt trauma than normal kidneys and may present with a history of disproportionate hematuria to the severity of trauma, being the most common renal abnormalities hydronephrosis, tumors and ectopic kidneys [45].

Hematuria may not be a reliable sign in children with renal trauma. In severe renal injuries 65% of children present gross hematuria and 33% microhematuria, this means that up to 2% of children with significant renal injuries present with no hematuria [43, 44].

Also the degree of hematuria does not correlate with the severity of the injury. Renal contusions may present with gross hematuria (31%), microhematuria (65%) or not hematuria

(3,4%) whereas severe injuries as complete ureteropelvic disruption or renal pedicle avulsions manifests with no hematuria [43, 44].

Due to these observations, hematuria alone cannot be used to decide which patients need further evaluation for renal trauma, it is important to consider the history of the injury, physical examination and clinical status. In children hypotension, on the other hand, is not a reliable indicator of the severity of the injury either. Many authors consider that children with a history of a significant deceleration or high-speed injury, significant external trauma and any degree of hematuria should undergo imaging regardless of blood presure. CT scan is the best imaging method to grade the severity of renal trauma. Children with minimal symptoms and microhematuria less than 50 RBCs/HPF may be observed without CT or screened with ultrasound [44].

Ureteral trauma is rare but ureteral injury due to blunt trauma is more common in children than in adults because a they are more flexible trunk and column. Hematuria is an ureliable sign and may be absent in 30-97% of cases.

If suspected, a delayed CT scan should be performed but the most sensitive diagnostic test is retrograde pyelogram (reserved if there are still doubts after CT) [43, 44].

Bladder at first ages is less protected because it has a higher position in the abdomen and thus is exposed above the pubis, the abdominal muscles are less developed and there is less abdominal fat to protect it.

Bladder traumatism is rare and it is usually associated with blunt trauma to a full bladder or pelvic fracture (though there is an increased incidence of bladder rupture in the absence of pelvic fracture compared to adults) [43, 44]. The main clinical signs are suprapubic pain, inability to void and hematuria. All patients with bladder injury have significant microhematuria and near 95% will show gross hematuria [43-47].

One third of bladder injuries are due to bladder contusion, it manifests with a variable degree of hematuria and it is treated with the placement of a urethral catheter until gross hematuria clears in most cases. Bladder ruptures may be intraperitoneal (more common in children because of the anatomic location of the bladder) which are usually managed by open surgical exploration, or extraperitoneal. Simple extraperitoneal bladder ruptures can be treated non-surgically with urethral catheter drainage. Bladder rupture can be diagnosed by a retrograde contrast filling of the bladder followed by radiography or CT scan [43-47].

Urethra in pediatric age is well protected and its damage is rare but urethral injury must be suspected in any patient with pelvic fracture o significant damage to the perineum. Signs of urethral injury are blood at the meatus, gross hematuria, pain at voiding or inability to void and there may be perineal and/or escrotal edema and hematoma. Management depends on the location and extension of the injury [43, 46].

1.6. Systemic or Autoinmune Disorders. Nephropathy

There are several nonsurgical disorders that may cause hematuria. Most of them have autoimmune response in common.

Acute poststreptococcal glomerulonephritis is the most common form of postinfectious nephritis worldwide. It is caused by immune damage to the glomeruli after postbacterial infection and may cause into pyelonephritis. Symptoms and signs usually appear several days

(2 to 3 weeks) after streptococcal group A, throat or skin infection. Clinical presentation includes the onset of hematuria (dark urine), edema, hypertension and proteinuria. The relationship between inflammation and arterial stiffness has been described. This phenomenon not only involves kidney, but also the arteries outside. This acute arterial stiffness might persist in patients who do not recover with a progression to either chronic renal insufficiency or end-stage renal disease [4, 48]. Diagnostic criteria include the evidence of streptococcal infection (positive group A streptococcal culture from skin or throat, or elevated anti-streptolysin O (ASO) (more common after pharyngeal infection but rarely after streptococcal skin infection) titre or anti-DNase B blood tests. Immune complex formation causes the decrease of C3 in acute phase and return to normal level after 6-8 weeks [48].

Renal biopsy should be considered in: acute renal failure, nephrotic syndrome, absence of evidence of streptococcal infection or persistence of lower C3 levels 2 months after the onset disease [48].

Treatment includes eradication of streptococcal infection by treatment of the acute disease that involves benzathine penicillin during 10 days and general measures like bed rest during the oliguric phase, diet, fluid balance, control of edema and hypertension. Early systemic antibiotic treatment for streptococcal throat or skin infection does not prevent the risk of glomerulonephritis. Complete recovery occurs in more than 95% of patients [4, 48].

Hemolytic-uremic syndrome is the most common cause of acute renal failure in children under 4 years of age. History of preceding gastroenteritis or acute upper respiratory infections a week before the onset of illness is usually presented. There is a heterogeneous group of phatogens like Shigella and Streptococcus pneumoniae, but the enterohaemorrhagic Escherichia coli-producing Shiga toxin O157:H7 is the most common infectious agent causing this syndrome [49].

This disease includes the triad of haemolytic anaemia, thrombocytopenia, and acute renal failure and also hepatosplenomegaly and hematuria. The primary event is the endotelial cell injury of capillary and arterial endotelium in the kidneys [49].

The majority of children with haemolytic uraemic syndrome develop some degree of renal insufficiency, and approximately two thirds of children will require dialysis therapy, while about one third will have milder renal involvement without the need of dialysis [49].

General management of acute renal failure includes appropriate fluid and electrolyte management, antihypertensive therapy, and the initiation of renal replacement therapy when appropriate. Specific management issues in this disease include treatment handling of the haematological complications, monitoring for extra-renal involvement, and avoiding antidiarrhoeal and antibiotic therapy. A new therapy for haemolytic uraemic syndrome is a humanised monoclonal antibody (Eculizumab) that blocks complement activity by cleavage of the complement protein C5 [49].

Disease prognosis depends on the proper management of acute renal failure. More than 90% of children survive the acute phase. End-stage renal disease may occur in about 9% of these patients [49].

Alport syndrome is a congenital x-linked dominant or autosomal recesive inherited abnormal collagen synthesis causing a functional defect in the glomerular basement membrane (lamellated glomerular basement membrane) and the inner ear. Patients may suffer from hematuria (that persists for at least a year), proteinuria and end-stage renal failure as a nephritis result, and also hearing loss, lenticonus, and retinal flecks [4, 50].

The diagnosis of Alport syndrome is suspected when an individual has glomerular hematuria or renal failure and a family history of Alport syndrome or renal failure without another obvious cause. Patients should undergo testing for microalbuminuria/ proteinuria as well as audiometry and ophthalmologic examination. Alport syndrome is confirmed showing a lamellated glomerular basement membrane at renal biopsy (glomerular collagen IV composition) and performing a genetic test where mutations in COL4A5, COL4A3 or COL4A4 are evidenced [50].

Treatment with angiotensin-converting enzyme inhibitors even before the onset of proteinuria, especially in individuals with genetic mutations or a family history consistent with early-onset renal failure, may delay the onset of end-stage disease and improve life expectancy [50].

Familial IgA disease (Immunoglobulin A nephropathy) is the most common form of idiopathic glomerulonephritis, and a substantial number of patients may succumb to end-stage renal disease. It is related to an accumulation of IgA immunoglobulin in the renal tisue [51]. Diagnosis is made by renal biopsy hystological examination. Diagnosis of this disease depends on the demonstration of mesangial IgA-dominant staining (by immunofluorescence or by immunohistochemistry). The clinical presentation of macroscopic hematuria is commonly provoked by upper respiratory tract infection or gastrointestinal disease. Some patients already have renal impairment, glomerular hematuria and hypertension at initial presentation [52].

Benign familial hematuria (thin basement membrane nephropathy) is a congenital autosomal dominant inherited disease and the most common cause of persistent hematuria in children and adults (affecting at least 1% of the population). The other main causes being IgA nephropathy and Alport síndrome [53].

Patients with benign familial hematuria present recurrent asymptomatic hematuria, while physical examination, laboratory tests (proteinuria, renal function) and urinary tract imaging are all normal.

Diagnosis is based on the fact that hematuria is found in other family members, and by ruling out other diseases. Also, patients have uniformly thinned glomerular basement membranes, as determined by electron microscopy [53].

At present, clinical diagnosis is still made mainly on the basis of persistent hematuria with minimal proteinuria and normal renal function, combined with electron microscopy examination and immunohistochemical evaluation of the type IV collagen-α-3 to α-5 chains. Immunohistochemical evaluation in renal biopsy has become a method of major importance in the differentiation between thin basement membrane nephropathy and early stages of Alport syndrome with microscopic hematuria. These collagen chains usually are either absent or abnormally distributed in Alport syndrome [53].

Benign familial hematuria is a lifelong nonprogressive disorder associated with family history [53].

Autosomal dominant / recesive polycystic kidney disease are important inherited kidney diseases with distinct clinical features and genetics.

Dominant pattern is the most common inherited kidney disease (1:1000) and afects both sexes equally [54]. Dominant polycystic kidney disease is a very rare case of end-stage renal disease in children. This pattern also includes not only polycystic kidneys but also abnormalities in other abdominal organs like liver, pancreas and intestinal tract and also in heart and vasculature. While the majority of these patients are diagnosed in adulthood, it is now well recognized that autosomal dominant polycystic kidney disease can be present in children of all ages [54].

Recessive polycystic kidney disease is rare (1:10.000/40.000) and the most severely affected infants may not survive. It afects both sexes equally. Recessive pattern primarily affects only two organs, kidney (polycystic kidneys) and liver (congenital hepatic fibrosis) [54].

These polycistic diseases are now termed "ciliopaties" because two of them share many important pathogenetic features related to the primary cilia such as abnormal cilia structure and/or function that involves kidney morphogenesis as well as the maintenance of the epitelial and endotelial layer [54].

Both polycystic kidney diseases are characterized by cystic dilatations of the renal tubules. In dominant disease, cysts can show massive expansion over time and can occur anywhere along the nephron. It is estimated that only 1% of nephrons become cystic [54].

In contrast recessive disease cysts are exclusively originated in collecting tubule, are generally much smaller (microcysts, not visible on gross examination) and all of the collecting tubules are causing fusiform dilatation radiating from cortex to medulla [54].

Alternatively to screening diagnosis finding in asymptomatic children, they may be diagnosed as part of an evaluation for gross hematuria or hypertension [4,54].

Other autoinmune diseases like *systemic lupus erythematosus* may cause hematuria, proteinuria and renal failure as a consequence of kidney damage. Treatment is based on immunosuppressive drugs and blood pressure control [4].

Henoch Schoenlein purpura is a non-thrombocytopenic systemic hypersensitivity vasculitis of childhood. Its etiology remains largely unknown, and the prognosis, depends primarily on the extent of renal involvement [55, 56]. The small blood vessel vasculitis is presented with petequial purpuric skin lesions, abdominal and joint pain, hematuria, and proteinuria. As many as 50% of patients may develop end-stage renal failure [4,55,56].

Renal involvement may manifest itself with haematuria, with or without proteinuria, and occasionally with nephritic or nephrotic syndrome, or with renal failure sometimes associated with a rapidly progressive glomerulonephritis. Although patients with only haematuria do not develop end-stage renal disease, those with proteinuria and haematuria may be associated with a 15% risk and the combination of nephritic-nephrotic syndrome with a 50% risk of progression to end-stage renal failure respectively. Treatment is based on steroids and pain control [55,56].

Hereditary hemorrhagic telangiectasia (Osler-Weber-Rendu disease) is a genetic (autosomal dominant) angiodysplasia affecting multiple organs. Clinical manifestations include spontaneous and recurrent epistaxis, mucocutaneous telangiectases that bleed easily and arteriovenous malformations in many organs. Renal arteriovenous fistulas and bladder, prostate and urethra telangiectases are reported to be among the causes of micro or macrohematuria associated to hereditary hemorrhagic telangiectasia [57].

1.7. Haematological Disorders

A bleeding disorder may present with hematuria. The obtention of a detailed familial history is mandatory because most of these disorders are inherited. Treatment is based on an accurate diagnosis of the disorder and correction of bleeding function [4].

Hematuria is one of the common signs in *sickle cell anemia*. Hematuria commonly occurs as a consequence of red blood cell sickling in the renal medulla, papillary necrosis, or even renal medullary carcinoma. Red blood cell sickling may obliterate small renal blood vessels leading to ischemia and hematuria. It is often accompanied by kidney pain [58].

Measures such as increased fluid ingestion, urine alkalinization and, if necessary, administration of epsilon-aminocaproic acid and certain invasive procedures have been proposed to treat hematuria. General measures such as preventive treatment manouvres like proper liquid intake and avoidance of exposure to cold are recommended [58].

Von Willebrand disease or von Willebrand factor-cleaving protease deficiency may cause micro or macro hematuria (mucosal bleeding). Von Willebrand deficiency is a complex disease where a quantitative and/or qualitative deficiency of von Willebrand factor is produced. This factor is a large glycoprotein essential for platelet adhesion and aggregation, especially at the high shear stress–associated hemodynamic conditions of the microcirculation. This factor allows primary hemostasis that mediates platelet plug formation via adhesion at the site of injury and protects FVIII in plasma from proteolytic degradation. Diagnosis of von Willebrand disease is based on von Willebrand antigen, factor (F) VIII clotting activity, and von Willebrand ristocetin cofactor activity determination [59, 60]

The most frequent symptoms in all patients were mucocutaneous ones: epistaxis (in 34% of children); prolonged bleeding from minor wounds (33%); and bruising (24%). Hematuria is less common. There are several standardized pediatric bleeding questionaries for the evaluation and follow-up of these patients which allow the detection of proper prophylactic hemostatic therapy [59, 60].

1.8. Induced by Drugs or Substancies

There are several drugs and sustancies that can cause hematuria at chilhood like toxins (gold, lead, mercury) that may trigger acute tubular necrosis. Drugs like penicillins, NSAIDs and penicillamine that provoke interstitial nephritis or cyclophosphamide, ritonavir and indinavir [61, 62].

1.9. Asimptomatic Micro-Macrohematuria. General Management

Asymptomatic gross or microscopic hematuria is relatively common in children. The prevalence of asymptomatic microscopic hematuria in scholar-age children has been estimated at 0.5% to 2.0%. The incidence of asymptomatic gross hematuria is estimated to be 0.13%. In more tan a half of the cases this is due to an easily identifiable cause. The clinical significance of asymptomatic hematuria is unclear [5]

Regarding microscopic hematuria, in 80% of cases there is no evidence about a particular etiology. Evaluation of redcell morphology might also be helpful in patients with hematuria. Redcells are typically uniform and round when there is extrarenal bleeding but they usually have a dysmorphic appearance in the presence of renal lesions, particularly glomerular disease [57].

The most frequent cause detect could be hypercalciuria in the abscense of stone disease (20% of these patients could have a family history of stone disease) followed by poststreptococcal glomerulonephritis (1%) resolved spontaneusly without complication [5]. This suggest that a diagnostic evaluation for posible causes of microscopic hematuria in children may not be necessary because asymptomatic microscopic hematuria in children is rarely associated with clinically important urinary tract disease and there are no longterm follow-up studies demonstrating that early detection of hypercalciuria is beneficial in preventing nephrolitiasis and bone demineralization [5,61]. In children with asymptomatic microscopic hematuria, radiological studies may fail to reveal abnormalities requiring clinical intervention. Thus, renal ultrasonography examination could be the only recommended study [5].

Table 2. Causes of red urine staining (discoloured urine)

Causes and agents that may color urine mimicking hematuria

-Myoglobin
-Urate crystals
-Free hemoglobin
-Porphyria
-Foods: red dyes in food, beets, blackberries
-Drugs: chloroquine,phenazopyridine,phenolphthalein, iron sorbitol, desferrioxamine

Rarely asymptomatic microscopic hematuria can be the first sign of occult renal disease. Normal renal biopsies or minor abnormalities were more frequently observed in several reports. However if this kind of hematuria occults glomerular disorders, progression to clinically significant disease will be accompained by the development of hypertension and/or proteinuria, thus long-term follow-up of these children performing anual urinalysis and blood presure measurement is mandatory [5,61,63,64].

On the other hand, a clinically important cause of asymptomatic gross hematuria could be much more common, despite of in 40% of cases no cause for the hematuria is ususally uncovered. The most frequent causes included hypercalciuria (as in microscopic hematuria), IgA nephropathy and post-streptococcal glomerulonephritis. As in microscopic hematuria, urinary tract infection was very rare cause [5,62].

Finally it is important to mention several causes that make red-brown urine discolouration that could mimic macroscopic hematuria situation [61,62, (table 2).

References

[1]   Grossfeld, G; Wolf Jr, J; Litwan, M; Hricak, H; Shuler, C; Agerter, D; Carroll, P. (2001). "Asymptomatic microscopic hematuria in adults: Summary of the AUA best practice policy recommendations". *American family physician,* 63(6), 1145–1154. PMID 11277551. edit

[2]   Greenfield, SP; Williot, P; Kaplan, D. Gross hematuria in children: a ten-year review. *Urology.*, 2007 Jan, 69(1), 166-9.

[3] Tu, WH; Shortliffe, LD. Evaluation of asymptomatic, atraumatic hematuria in children and adults. Nat Rev Urol. 2010 Apr;7(4):189-94. doi: 10.1038/nrurol.2010.27. Epub 2010 Mar 9.

[4] Halachmi, S; Kakiashvili, D; Meretyk, S. A review on hematuria in children. *ScientificWorldJournal.*, 2006 Mar, 8, 6, 311-7.

[5] Bergstein, J; Leiser, J; Andreoli, S. The clinical significance of asymptomatic gross and microscopic hematuria in children. *Arch Pediatr Adolesc Med.*, 2005 Apr, 159(4), 353-5.

[6] Bergstein, J; Leiser, J; Andreoli, S. The clinical significance of asymptomatic gross and microscopic hematuria in children. *Arch Pediatr Adolesc Med.*, 2005 Apr, 159(4), 353-5.

[7] Molimard, B; Al-Qahtani, S; Lakmichi, A; Sejiny, M; Gil-Diez de Medina, S; Carpentier, X; Traxer, O. Flexible ureterorenoscopy with holmium laser in horseshoe kidneys. *Urology.*, 2010 Dec, 76(6), 1334-7. doi: 10.1016/j.urology.2010.02.072. Epub 2010 Jun 22. Review.

[8] Gorospe, EC; Aigbe, MO. Nutcracker syndrome: a rare cause of hematuria. *ScientificWorldJournal.*, 2006 Jun, 30, 6, 745-6.

[9] Rudloff, U; Holmes, RJ; Prem, JT; Faust, GR; Moldwin, R; Siegel, D. Mesoaortic compression of the left renal vein (nutcracker syndrome): case reports and review of the literature. *Ann Vasc Surg.*, 2006 Jan, 20(1), 120-9.

[10] Loghman-Adham, M1; Tejero, HT; London, R. Acute hemorrhagic cystitis due to Escherichia coli. *Child Nephrol Urol.*, 1988-1989, 9(1-2), 29-32.

[11] Mufson, MA; Belshe, RB. A review of adenoviruses in the etiology of acute hemorrhagic cystitis. *J Urol.*, 1976 Feb, 115(2), 191-4.

[12] Decker, DB; Karam, JA; Wilcox, DT. Pediatric hemorrhagic cystitis. *J Pediatr Urol.*, 2009 Aug, 5(4), 254-64. doi: 10.1016/j.jpurol.2009.02.199. Epub 2009 Mar 19.

[13] Hatakeyama, N; Suzuki, N; Yamamoto, M; Kuroiwa, Y; Hori, T; Mizue, N; Tsutsumi H. Detection of BK virus and adenovirus in the urine from children after allogeneic stem cell transplantation. *Pediatr Infect Dis J.*, 2006 Jan, 25(1), 84-5.

[14] Mori, Y; Miyamoto, T; Kato, K; Kamezaki, K; Kuriyama, T; Oku, S; Takenaka, K; Iwasaki, H; Harada, N; Shiratsuchi, M; Abe, Y; Nagafuji, K; Teshima, T; Akashi, K. Different risk factors related to adenovirus- or BK virus-associated hemorrhagic cystitis following allogeneic stem cell transplantation. *Biol Blood Marrow Transplant.*, 2012 Mar, 18(3), 458-65. doi: 10.1016/j.bbmt.2011.07.025. Epub 2011 Jul 31.

[15] Vögeli, TA; Peinemann, F; Burdach, S; Ackermann, R. Urological treatment and clinical course of BK polyomavirus-associated hemorrhagic cystitis in children after bone marrow transplantation. *Eur Urol.*, 1999 Sep, 36(3), 252-7.

[16] Cipe, FE; Soygür, T; Doğu, F; Erdoğan, O; Bozdoğan, G; Ikincioğullari, A. Late onset hemorrhagic cystitis in a hematopoietic stem cell recipient: treatment with intravesical hyaluronic acid. *Pediatr Transplant.*, 2010 Sep 1, 14(6), E79-82. doi: 10.1111/j.1399-3046.2009.01169.x. Epub 2009 Apr 1.

[17] Miodosky, M; Abdul-Hai, A; Tsirigotis, P; Or, R; Bitan, M; Resnick, IB; Gesundheit, B; Zilberman, I; Ioffe, L; Leubovic, A; Slavin, S; Shapira, MY. Treatment of post-hematopoietic stem cell transplantation hemorrhagic cystitis with intravesicular sodium hyaluronate. Bone Marrow Transplant., 2006 Oct, 38(7), 507-11.

[18] Young, G; Toretsky, JA; Campbell, AB; Eskenazi, AE. Recognition of common

childhood malignancies. *Am Fam Physician.*, 2000 Apr 1, 61(7), 2144-54.

[19] Leung, RS; Liesner, R; Brock, P. Coagulopathy as a presenting feature of Wilms tumour. *Eur J Pediatr.* 2004 Jul, 163(7), 369-73. Epub 2004 Apr 8.

[20] Raney, B; Anderson, J; Jenney, M; Arndt, C; Brecht, I; Carli, M; Bisogno, G; Oberlin, O; Rey, A; Treuner, J; Ullrich, F; Stevens, M. Late effects in 164 patients with rhabdomyosarcoma of the bladder/prostate region: a report from the international workshop. *J Urol.*, 2006 Nov, 176(5), 2190-4; discussion 2194-5.

[21] Rosenberg, HK; Eggli, KD; Zerin, JM; Ortega, W; Wallach, MT; Kolberg, H; Lebowitz RL; Snyder, HM. Benign cystitis in children mimicking rhabdomyosarcoma. *J Ultrasound Med.*, 1994 Dec, 13(12), 921-32.

[22] Kojima, S; Yagi M; Asagiri, K; Fukahori, S; Tanaka, Y; Ishii, S; Saikusa, N; Koga, Y; Yoshida, M; Masui, D; Komatsuzaki, N; Nakagawa, S; Ozono, S; Tanikawa, K. Infantile neuroblastoma of the urinary bladder detected by hematuria. *Pediatr Surg Int.*, 2013 Jul, 29(7), 753-7. doi: 10.1007/s00383-013-3305-9. Epub 2013 Mar 31.

[23] Heinzelmann, F; Thorwarth, D; Lamprecht, U; Kaulich, TW; Fuchs, J; Seitz, G; Ebinger, M; Handgretinger, R; Bamberg, M; Weinmann, M. Comparison of different adjuvant radiotherapy approaches in childhood bladder/prostate rhabdomyosarcoma treated with conservative surgery. *Strahlenther Onkol.*, 2011 Nov, 187(11), 715-21.

[24] Lerena, J; Krauel, L; García-Aparicio, L; Vallasciani, S; Suñol, M; Rodó, J. Transitional cell carcinoma of the bladder in children and adolescents: six-case series and review of the literatura. *J Pediatr Urol.*, 2010 Oct, 6(5), 481-5

[25] Gülpinar, O; Soygür, T; Baltaci, S; Akand, M; Kankaya, D. Transitional cell carcinoma of bladder with lamina propria invasion in a 10-year-old boy. *Urology.*, 2006 Jul, 68(1), 204.e1-3.

[26] Takemoto, J; Yamazaki, Y; Sakai, K. A case of large bladder hemangioma successfully treated with endoscopic yttrium aluminium garnet laser irradiation. *Int J Urol.*, 2011 Dec, 18(12), 854-6.

[27] March Villalba, JA; Domínguez Hinarejos, C; Serrano Durbá, A; García Ibarra, F. Bladder cavernous hemangioma as a cause of hematuria in a child. *Actas Urol Esp.*, 2010 Mar, 34(3), 299-301.

[28] Bohn, OL; Pardo-Castillo, E; Fuertes-Camilo, M; Rios-Luna, NP; Martinez, A; Sanchez-Sosa, S. Urinary bladder paraganglioma in childhood: a case report and review of the literature. *Pediatr Dev Pathol.*, 2011 Jul-Aug, 14(4), 327-32.

[29] Türk, C; Knoll, T; Petrik, A; Sarica, K; Skolarikos, A; Straub, M; Seitz, C. Guidelines on Urolithiasis. Uroweb 2013. Available at: http://www.uroweb.org/gls/pdf/ 21_Urolithiasis_LRV4.pdf

[30] Straub, M; Strohmaier, WL; Berg, W; Beck, B; Hoppe, B; Laube, N; Lahme, S; Schmidt, M; Hesse, A; Koehrmann, KU. Diagnosis and metaphylaxis of stone disease. Consensus concept of the National Working Committee on Stone Disease for the upcoming German Urolithiasis Guideline. *World J Urol*, 2005, 23, 309-23.

[31] Valentini, RP; Lakshmanan, Y. Nephrolithiasis in children. *Adv Chronic Kidney Dis*, 2011, 18, 370-5.

[32] Matlaga, BR; Schaeffer, AJ; Novak, TE; Trock, BJ. Epidemiologic insights into pediatric kidney stone disease. *Urol Res*, 2010, 38, 453-7.

[33] Tekgül, S; Riedmiller, H; Dogan, HS; Hoebeke, P; Kocvara, R; Nijman, R; Radmayr Chr; Stein, R. Guidelines on Paediatric Urology. *Uroweb*, 2013. Available at:

http://www.uroweb.org/gls/pdf/22%20Paediatric%20Urology_LR.pdf

[34] Elmacı, AM; Ece, A; Akın, F. Clinical characteristics and metabolic abnormalities in preschool-age children with urolithiasis in southeast Anatolia. *J Pediatr Urol*, 2013, http://dx.doi.org/10.1016/j.jpurol.2013.11.004

[35] Milošević, D; Batinić, D; Turudić, D; Batinić, D; Topalović-Grković, M; Gradiški, IP. Demographic characteristics and metabolic risk factors in Croatian children with urolithiasis. *Eur J Pediatr*, 2014, 173, 353-9.

[36] Bove, P; Kaplan, D; Dalrymple, N; Rosenfield, AT; Verga, M; Anderson, K; Smith, RC. Reexamining the value of hematuria testing in patients with acute flank pain. *J Urol*, 1999, 162, 685-7.

[37] Persaud, AC; Stevenson, MD; McMahon, DR; Christopher, NC. Pediatric urolithiasis: clinical predictors in the emergency department. Pediatrics, 2009, 124, 888-94.

[38] Moghtaderi, M; Noohi, AH; Safaeyan, B; Abbasi, A; Sabsechian, M; Meherkash, M. Screening for microscopic hematuria in school-age children of Gorgan City. *Iran J Kidney Dis*, 2014, 8, 70-2.

[39] Sternberg, K; Greenfield, SP; Williot, P; Wan, J. Pediatric stone disease: an evolving experience. *J Urol*, 2005, 174, 1711-4.

[40] Dursun, I; Poyrazoglu, HM; Dusunsel, R; Gunduz, Z; Gurgoze, MK; Demirci, D; Kucukaydin, M. Pediatric urolithiasis: an 8-year experience of single centre. *Int Urol Nephrol*, 2008, 40, 3-9.

[41] Alpay, H; Ozen, A; Gokce, I; Biyikli, N. Clinical and metabolic features of urolithiasis and microlithiasis in children. *Pediatr Nephrol*, 2009, 24, 2203-9.

[42] Sternberg, K; Greenfield, SP; Williot, P; Wan, J. Pediatric stone disease: an evolving experience. *J Urol.*, 2005 Oct,174(4 Pt 2), 1711-4

[43] Sarica, K. Pediatric urolithiasis: etiology, specific pathogenesis and medical treatment. *Urol Res*, 2006, 34, 96-101

[44] Tegül, S; Riedmiller, H; Dogan, HS; Hoebeke, P; Kocvara, Nijman, R; Radmayr, Chr; Stein, R. EAU Guidelines on Paediatric Urology. European Society for Paediatric Urology. *European Association of Urology*, 2013.

[45] Casale, JA. Urinary Tract Trauma. In Gearhart et al. *Paediatric Urology*. 2nd edition. Philadelphia: *Saunders Elsevier*, 2010. ISBN: 978-1-4160-3204-5. pp 720-736.

[46] Husmann, AD. Upper urinary tract trauma. In *The Kelalis-King-Belman Textbook of Clinical Pediatric Urology*. 5th edition. UK: informa healthcare, 2007. ISBN 13: 978 1 84184 504 3. pp 529-537.

[47] Pichler, R; Fritsch, H; Skradski, V; Horninger, W; Schlenck, B; Rehder, P; Oswald J. Diagnosis and management of pediatric urethral injuries. *Urol Int.*, 2012, 89(2), 136-42.

[48] Yu, MC; Yu, MS; Yu, MK; Lee, F; Huang, WH. Acute reversible changes of brachial-ankle pulse wave velocity in children with acute poststreptococcal glomerulonephritis. *Pediatr Nephrol.*, 2011 Feb, 26(2), 233-9.

[49] Scheiring, J; Rosales, A; Zimmerhackl, LB. Clinical practice. Today's understanding of the haemolytic uraemic syndrome. *Eur J Pediatr.*, 2010 Jan, 169(1), 7-13.

[50] Savige, J; Gregory, M; Gross, O; Kashtan, C; Ding, J; Flinter, F. Expert guidelines for the management of Alport syndrome and thin basement membrane nephropathy. *J Am Soc Nephrol.*, 2013 Feb, 24(3), 364-75. doi: 10.1681/ASN.2012020148. Epub 2013 Jan 24.

[51] Goto, M; Wakai, K; Kawamura, T; Ando, M; Endoh, M; Tomino, Y. A scoring system

to predict renal outcome in IgA nephropathy: a nationwide 10-year prospective cohort study. *Nephrol Dial Transplant.* 2009 Oct;24(10), 3068-74. doi: 10.1093/ndt/gfp273. Epub 2009 Jun 10.

[52]   Maixnerová, D; Tesař, V; Ryšavá, R; Reiterová, J; Poupětová, H; Dvořáková, L; Goláň, L; Neprašová, M; Kidorová, J; Merta, M; Honsová, E. The coincidence of IgA nephropathy and Fabry disease. *BMC Nephrol.*, 2013 Jan 11;14, 6. doi: 10.1186/1471-2369-14-6.

[53]   Tryggvason, K; Patrakka, J. Thin basement membrane nephropathy. *J Am Soc Nephrol.*, 2006 Mar, 17(3), 813-22. Epub 2006 Feb 8.

[54]   Dell, KM. The spectrum of polycystic kidney disease in children. *Adv Chronic Kidney Dis.*, 2011 Sep, 18(5), 339-47

[55]   Narchi, H. Risk of long term renal impairment and duration of follow up recommended for Henoch-Schonlein purpura with normal or minimal urinary findings: a systematic review. *Arch Dis Child.*, 2005 Sep, 90(9), 916-20. Epub 2005 May 4.

[56]   Chen, O; Zhu, XB; Ren, P; Wang, YB; Sun, RP; Wei, DE. Henoch Schonlein Purpura in children: clinical analysis of 120 cases. *Afr Health Sci.*, 2013 Mar, 13(1), 94-9.

[57]   Di Gennaro, L; Ramunni, A; Suppressa, P; Guastamacchia, E; Resta, F; Sabbà, C. Asymptomatic microhematuria: an indication of hereditary hemorrhagic telangiectasia? J Urol. 2005 Jan,173(1), 106-9.

[58]   de Santis Feltran, L1; de Abreu Carvalhaes, JT; Sesso, R. Renal complications of sickle cell disease: managing for optimal outcomes. *Paediatr Drugs.*, 2002, 4(1), 29-36.

[59]   Berber E. The Molecular Genetics of von Willebrand Disease. *Turk J Haematol.*, 2012 Dec, 29(4), 313-324.

[60]   Biss, TT; Blanchette, VS; Clark, DS; Bowman, M; Wakefield, CD; Silva, M; Lillicrap D; James, PD; Rand, ML. Quantitation of bleeding symptoms in children with von Willebrand disease: use of a standardized pediatric bleeding questionnaire. *J Thromb Haemost.*, 2010 May, 8(5), 950-6.

[61]   Phadke, KD; Vijayakumar, M; Sharma, J; Iyengar, A. Indian Pediatric Nephrology Group. Consensus statement on evaluation of hematuria. Indian Pediatr. 2006 Nov, 43(11), 965-73.

[62]   Gattineni, J. Highlights for the management of a child with proteinuria and hematuria. *Int J Pediatr.*, 2012, 2012, 768142

[63]   Feng, CY; Xia, YH; Wang, WJ; Xia, J; Fu, HD; Wang, X; Shen, HJ; Qian, GL; Liu, AM; Mao, JH. Persistent asymptomatic isolated hematuria in children: clinical and histopathological features and prognosis. *World J Pediatr.* 2013 May, 9(2), 163-8.

[64]   Kovacević, Z; Jovanović, D; Rabrenović, V; Dimitrijević, J; Djukanović J. Asymptomatic microscopic haematuria in young males. *Int J Clin Pract.*, 2008 Mar, 62(3), 406-12.

In: Hematuria
Editors: Nikhil Vasdev and G. Boustead

ISBN: 978-1-63463-073-3
© 2015 Nova Science Publishers, Inc.

Chapter 12

Haematuria Secondary to Benign Prostatic Hyperplasia

Nikhil Vasdev[1], Katherine James[1], Tim Lane[1], James M. Adshead[1],
Gregory Boustead[1] and Andrew C. Thorpe[2]*

[1]Hertfordshire and South Bedfordshire Urological Cancer Centre,
Department of Urology, Lister Hospital, Stevenage, UK
[2]Department of Urology, Freeman Hospital, Newcastle upon Tyne, UK

Haematuria is common clinical presentation with a community prevalence of 1 in 40 patients [1] and is estimated to account for 4 - 20% of all urological hospital visits [2]. The gradual rise in patient referrals to urological clinics is attributed to the increased use of urine dipstick analysis in the community [3]. Current recommendations from the Department of Health, United Kingdom presume that occult pathology may be present following haematuria presentation and as such should be investigated4. Further studies advocate urgent investigations of haematuria via a 'Fast-track one-stop haematuria clinic' [4].

Common causes of haematuria in men include urinary infection, urological malignancy and benign prostatic hyperplasia (BPH). The latter diagnosis often results in vascular enlargement of the prostate leading to haematuria. In clinical practice, these patients present at a designated haematuria clinic resulting in extensive investigations. Variations exist within the literature as to the proportion of patients with normal investigations. Khadra et al. [5] quoted a no diagnosis rate of 56.6% in males whilst Edwards et al. suggested a higher rate of 76.7%.

Treatment for BPH involves medical or surgical management options. A Trans-urethral resection of the prostate (TURP) is the one of most common types of surgical management offered. However, despite this intervention patients can re-present with further haematuria following a TURP. Often, this results in further clinical assessment at the Haematuria clinic, which escalates the economic burden and patient anxiety following haematuria investigation. Murakami et al. [6] suggested that if patients with persistent haematuria are followed then a

---

* Correspondence – nikhilvasdev@doctors.org.uk.

significant proportion will be shown to have undiscovered neoplasia. However, Khadra et al. suggested that if the initial investigation was thorough then the chance of missing significant pathology is small. Furthermore, some studies have suggested that prolonged bleeding can result in haematuria in otherwise normal patients [7,8]. Others have suggested anti-coagulant therapy may result in haematuria in as many as 40% of cases [8].

There are two main groups of patients who present with haematuria secondary to BPH. The first group includes those patients who have a vascular BPH and the second are those who have a re-bleed following a previous TURP due to a vascular re-growth of the prostate.

We have recently published on this subjected [9]. In our study we retrospectively archived the data of 166 men diagnosed with hematuria secondary to BPH from our hematuria clinic database from March 2003 and March 2006. The 166 patients were divided into 2 groups: Group I (n = 94) hematuria with no previous TURP; Group II (n = 72) hematuria with previous TURP. The clinical management in both groups included reassurance, commencement of a 5-alpha reductase inhibitor (finasteride) or a primary TURP in Group I or re-do TURP in Group II. Results: The median age was 73 years (range 45–94 years) for both groups. Outcomes combined for both groups included: reassurance alone in 26% (n = 43), finasteride in 51% (n = 84) and TURP in 12% (n = 19). Patients managed with reassurance alone or TURP had no further episodes of hematuria. At a mean follow-up was 18 months (range 7–22 months), 2 patients treated with finasteride re-bled but did require further intervention.

A further 2 men elected to stop finasteride due to erectile dysfunction and gynecomastia respectively. We concluded that BPH can present with hematuria. Following re-evaluation in a hematuria clinic, the lack of any subsequent cancer diagnosis in these patients suggests that repeat hematuria investigations should be carefully re-considered [9].

On the basis of current literature and our experience we can conclude the following for patients with haematuria secondary to BPH

1. Causes of haematuria in men include urinary infection, urological malignancy and prostatic enlargement in the form of Benign Prostatic Hyperplasia (BPH). Vascular enlargement of the prostate often leads to haematuria in male patients. In clinical practice, these patients present at the haematuria clinic and following extensive investigations treatment in the form of medical or surgical management is offered. We therefore aimed to identify any differences in clinical assessment outcomes between male patients, presenting with haematuria, pre- and post-TURP. We hypothesised that BPH patients - re-presenting with haematuria following a TURP - do not warrant further investigation as this rarely provides any new pathology resulting in further treatment

2. BPH can re-present with further haematuria. Conservative treatment options include reassurance and 5-α Reductase inhibitors such as Finasteride. Surgical options for persistent haematuria with LUTS can be managed by TURP. The lack of any cancer diagnoses in this cohort of patients suggests that repeat haematuria investigations of flexible cystoscopy and imaging are not necessarily required. On the basis of latest clinical evidence we propose that invasive and more expensive investigations should only be undertaken if the clinical picture appears suspicious.

References

[1] Ritchie CD, Bevan EA, Collier SJ. Importance of occult haematuria found at screening. *Br. Med. J. (Clin. Res. Ed) 1986* ; 292: 681-683.

[2] Mariani AJ, Mariani MC, Macchioni C, Stams UK, Hariharan A, Moriera A. The significance of adult hematuria: 1,000 hematuria evaluations including a risk-benefit and cost-effectiveness analysis. *J. Urol. 1989* ;141(2):350-5.

[3] Edwards TJ, Dickinson AJ, Natale S, Gosling J, McGrath JS. A prospective analysis of the diagnostic yield resulting from the attendance of 4020 patients at a protocol-driven haematuria clinic. *BJU Int. 2006* Feb;97(2):301-5.

[4] Department of health. Guidelines for Urgent Referrals of Patients with Suspected Cancers. London: Department of Health, 2004.

[5] Khadra MH, Pickard RS, Charlton M, Powell PH, Neal DE. A prospective analysis of 1,930 patients with hematuria to evaluate current diagnostic practice. *J. Urol. 2000 Feb*;163(2):524-7.

[6] Murakami S, Igarashi T, Hara S et al. Strategies for asymptomatic microscopic hematuria: a prospective study of 1034 patients. *J. Urol.* 1990; 144:99.

[7] Kraus SF, Siroky MB, Babyan R et al. Hematuria and the use of non-steroidal anti-inflammatory drugs. *J. Urol.* 1984;132:288.

[8] Benton O, Lazarchick J, Orak JK et al. Use of a bleeding time determination in the evaluation of unexplained hematuria. *J. Urol.* 1987; 137:527.

[9] Vasdev N, A Kumar, Verrtapillay R, Thorpe AC. Haematuria secondary to benign prostatic hyperplasia - retrospective analysis of 166 men identified in a single one stop haematuria clinic. *Current Urology* 2012;6;93-98.

In: Hematuria
Editors: Nikhil Vasdev and G. Boustead

ISBN: 978-1-63463-073-3
© 2015 Nova Science Publishers, Inc.

Chapter 13

Haematuria and Bladder Cancer: Definition, Diagnosis, Management and Prognosis

*Nikhil Vasdev**

Hertfordshire and South Bedfordshire Urological Cancer Centre,
Department of Urology, Lister Hospital, Stevenage, UK

Introduction

Haematuria is defined as the presence of the blood in urine. However, the Joint Consensus Statement on the Initial Assessment of Haematuria that was prepared jointly by the Renal Association recently published the definition of 'Haematuria' in the UK and the British Association of Urological Surgeons published in 2008. According to this document [1] blood in the urine either visible i.e., gross or macroscopic or non-visible haematuria. The non-visible haematuria is classified into symptomatic visible haematuria or asymptomatic non-visible haematuria. Symptomatic haematuria is haematuria that is associated with patient symptoms such as pain or lower urinary tract symptoms. Asymptomatic haematuria is associated with no symptoms.

Definition

The definition of non-visible haematuria is different as per different international guidelines. The American Urological Association (AUA guidelines) define non visible haematuria as >3 RBC s per high power field on a spun specimen, Nephrologist defined non visible haematuria as > 5 RBCs per microliter, JAMA (Journal of the American Medical

---
* Correspondence nikhilvasdev@doctors.org.uk.

Association) as > 2-3 RBC per high powered field and Campbell Walsh definition of non visible haematuria being > 5 per high powered field for spun urine and > 2 RBC's per high powered field of unspun urine.

The diagnosis of non-visible haematuria especially asymptomatic non-visible haematuria is on the basis of a dipstick analysis. The urine dipstick analysis for blood is confirmed via the chromogen indicator on the dipstick, orthotolidine that is a peroxidise substrate. When haemoglobin, which contains peroxidise activity come in contact with orthotolidine, an oxidation reaction commences that results in the colour change to blue of the indicator. It is very important to be aware of the false positive results that can occur with a dipstick analysis with regards to non-visible haematuria in order to prevent the ordering of unnecessary investigations. False positive results can occur due to the presence of oxidising agents in the urine from exercise, dehydration, menstrual blood, povine iodine and hypochlorite solutions such as bleech. False negatives can occur due to the presence of reducing agents such as vitamin C, gentisic acid and poorly mixed urine.

In addition to urine dipstick analysis as mentioned above can have a false positive result. In order to minimize the risk electronic strip readers are used to overcome this. Despite this it is very important to remember that there is no substitution for urine microscopy performed in a regulated component laboratory.

In the United Kingdom there are guidelines to determine the degree of positively. With regards to dipstick versus microscopy diagnosis, it is important to ensure that the Urine dipstick of a fresh voided urine sample, containing no preservative, is considered a sensitive means of detecting the presence of haematuria. When patients are seen in outpatient clinics it is common for patient to carry urine into the clinic in a clean jar from home. This may results in an increase in the community based urine samples sent for microscopy have a significant false negative rate; the procedure is more labour intensive, and adds little to establishing the diagnosis of haematuria. Routine microscopy for confirmation of dipstick haematuria is not necessary.

When a urine result from a dipstick is reported as a "Trace" it is important to know the difference between a "Trace" versus "1+". Whilst the sensitivity of urine dipsticks may vary from one manufacturer to another, significant haematuria is considered to be 1+ or greater. Trace haematuria should be considered negative.

In certain situations Haemolysed versus non-haemolysed urine dipstick results are reported. It has been found that there is no distinction in significance between non-haemolysed and haemolysed dipstick-positive haematuria. 1+ positive for either should be considered of equal significance.

The next question is who should be investigated for haematuria as against discharging the patient. To address this question the BAUS [1] guidelines help define patients with "significant haematuria". These patients are those who have had a single episode of visible haematuria, any single episode of symptomatic non-visible haematuria in the absence of a urinary tract infection or a possible transient cause or in a patient with persistent asymptomatic non-visible haematuria. Persistent asymptomatic non-visible haematuria is defined as the presence of 2 out of 3 dipsticks positive for non-visible haematuria.

Prior to proceeding to investigations for haematuria it is important to evaluate and exclude both transient causes and false positive cause of non-visible haematuria. The commonest transient cause is a urinary tract infection, exercise or menstruation [2].

In the UK most of these patient are seen in an urgent single investigation clinic called the "One stop haematuria clinic". The patients who are prioritized as urgent referrals in the "One stop haematuria clinic" are referred in as urgent "2 week wait rules". These patients include all patients with visible haematuria (any age), all patients with symptomatic non-visible haematuria (any age) and all patients with asymptomatic non-visible haematuria aged ≥40 yrs. In "One stop haematuria clinic" patients are reviewed and detailed history and examination is performed. Examination includes abdominal, genital and a digital rectal examination in men to evaluate the prostate. In women a per-vaginal examination is performed specially in the elderly female population to exclude vaginal examination. A urine culture is performed but there is debate on the role of performing urine cytology in all patients. In patient with symptomatic non visible haematuria or persistent asymptomatic non visible haematuria specific investigations performed include a plasma creatinine/eGFR, proteinuria on dipstick and a blood pressure To measure proteinuria on a random sample a urine for protein:creatinine ratio (PCR) oralbumin:creatinine ratio (ACR) on a random sample (according to local practice). An ultrasound of the renal tract is preformed in patients with non-visible haematuria and a CT-Urogram in patients with visible haematuria. All patients have a flexible cystoscopy performed the same day.

In those patients in whom a urological cause has been excluded a nephrology referral is made. The need for a nephrology referral in this situation depends on factors other than simply the presence of haematuria. The UK NICE chronic kidney disease guidelines for such referral criteria will be published in September 2008. Nephrology referral is recommended if there is concurrent evidence of declining GFR (by >10ml/min at any stage within the previous 5 years or by >5ml/min within the last 1 year) or in the presence of Stage 4 or 5 CKD (eGFR <30ml/min), significant proteinuria (ACR ≥30mg/mmol or PCR ≥50mg/mmol) , Isolated haematuria (i.e., in the absence of significant proteinuria) with hypertension in those aged <40 or Visible haematuria coinciding with intercurrent (usually upper respiratory tract) infection .

The evidence for investigating patients with haematuria comes from two UK studies the first was by Khadra et al. [3] and second from Edwards et al. [4]. In Khardra et al. [3] study a total of 1,930 patients were enrolled prospectively in the study at a haematuria clinic between October 1994 and March 1997. Evaluation consisted of basic demographics, history and examination, routine blood tests, urinalysis and cytology. All patients underwent plain abdominal radiography, renal ultrasound, IVP and flexible cystoscopy. Data showed that total of 1,194 males and 736 females with a mean age of 58 years (range 17 to 96) were included in the study. Overall, 61% of patients had no basis found for haematuria, 12% had bladder cancer, 13% had urinary tract infection and 2% had stones. Kidney and upper tract tumours were noted in 14 patients (0.7%), including 4 who presented with microscopic haematuria. If only ultrasound or IVP had been performed 4 of these cases would have been missed. Of 982 patients presenting with microscopic haematuria 51 had cancer. Bladder cancer was found in 7 patients younger than 40 years. In total 61% of the cohort had no pathology detected. In the remainder of the patients, 12% had a diagnosis of bladder cancer, 13% had a proven urinary tract infection and 2% had stone disease. The main message of this paper was that if only an ultrasound or intravenous urogram were used, four patients with an upper urinary tract malignancy would have been missed hence the paper recommended performing both an ultrasound and Intravenous urogram in patients with haematuria. The overall incidence of a diagnosis of a urological malignancy was 24% in this paper and 5% of patients with non-visible haematuria had a diagnosis of bladder cancer confirmed.

The second paper by Edwards et al. [4] was a larger study of 4020 patients attending between October 1998 and August 2003. All patient had an ultrasound of kidneys and a flexible cystoscopy. Subsequently, Intravenous Urogram was used where indicated following abnormal first-line tests and in patients with persistent haematuria where no abnormality had been detected. The authors found 2627 men and 1393 women presented with microscopic (53.2%) or macroscopic haematuria (46.8%). The overall prevalence of malignant disease was 12.1%, but for macroscopic haematuria it was 18.9% and for microscopic haematuria 4.8%. Age and sex also influenced the observed rates of disease. Of the upper tract tumours, 70 were identified after abnormal US, with three cases of transitional cell carcinoma identified on IVU after a normal US. In patients with visible haematuria the patients had a four-fold increase in the diagnosis of cancer compared with non visible haematuria (18.9% versus 4.8%). In this study the incidence of negative pathology on investigations was 75%. Three patients with an upper tract tumour were identified after normal ultrasounds scan on an intravenous urogram.

Haematuria and Bladder Cancer

Once a patient has had a diagnosis of bladder lesion detected on flexible cystoscopy they are subsequently placed on the urgent operating list for Trans-urethral resection of bladder tumour (TURBT). Most centres in the UK perform a white light cystoscopy but there is now a gradual increase in the number of centres performing fluorescence cystosocpy.

When a patient is placed on the operative list for TURBT, the consent form must cover potential side effects of the procedure including the risk of bleeding, infection and bladder perforation. The patients should also be told about the role of mitomycin C (MMC) that is given post operatively within 6-24 hours in the UK in order to prevent recurrence.

On commencing a TURBT the patient either has a general or spinal anaesthetic. If the tumour is located on the lateral wall there is a risk of an intraoperative obturator kick that can result in an ontable perforation. The patient in this case should be paralyzed with a muscle relaxant. A TURBT involves the examination of the bladder initially with a 30 degree and 70 degree cystoscope. A bimanual examination is performed at the same time of the cystoscopy (Figure 1). A 26 Fr or 28 Fr Resectoscope is introduced a resection of the bladder tumour is performed using monopolar diathermy to resect the exophytic region of the tumour followed by the resection of deep resection biopsies from the base of the tumour. On the completion of the resection and securing haemostasis with a roller ball diathermy a catheter is placed insitu. The specimen is then sent for histological analysis. There are some very important principals in performing a thorough TURBT which include that the procedure is initiated with careful bimanual palpation under general or spinal anaesthesia; Insertion of the resectoscope, in men under visual guidance, with inspection of the whole urethra; Inspection of the whole urothelial lining of the bladder; biopsy from prostatic urethra if indicated: Cold-cup bladder biopsies if indicated and Resection of the tumour.

There are a few units in the UK that are performing fluorescent cystoscopy either with a photodynamic diagnosis (PDD) or blue light cystoscopy, which is performed using the handling of, 5-ALA (5-Aminolevulinic Acid) by the tumour. The mechanism of action of 5-ALA for patients with bladder cancer is related to the installation of 5-ALA pre-cystoscopy. The 5-ALA is taken up by the urothelium and converted to protoporphyrin, which is preferentially. When a blue light cystoscope is used with a wavelength of 375 – 440 nm this leads on to a higher intensity illumination of the abnormal mucosa compared with surrounding normal mucosa. This in clinical practice has lead to a 30% increase in the diagnosis of bladder cancer and a 67% in the diagnosis of carcinoma in situ of the bladder [5].

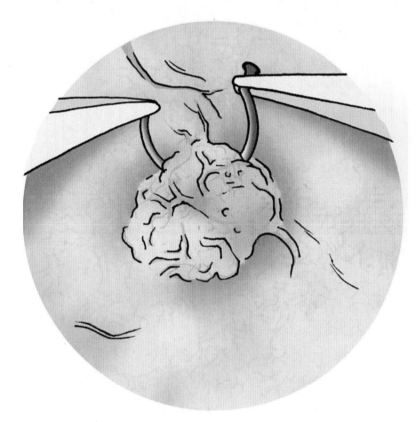

Figure 1. A Transurethral resection of bladder tumour.

When a patient has had a TURBT the specimen is sent for histological analysis it is staged as per the 2009 TNM classification of urinary bladder cancer [6] [Table 1]. Tumours that have invaded the lamina propria are classified as stage T1. Ta and T1 tumours can be removed by transurethral resection (TURBT), and therefore they are grouped under the heading of NMIBC for therapeutic purposes. T2 disease stage and above is classified into muscle invasive bladder cancer. Also included under this heading are flat, high-grade tumours that are confined to the mucosa, and classified as CIS (Tis). The World health organization (WHO) system grades tumours of the bladder into a 1973 or 2004 classification. Most patients in the UK receive post operatively will receive intravesical Mitomycin-C (MMC). Mitomycin C is an anti-tumour antibiotic that has anti-tumour activity by cross linking complementary DNA strands and alkylates single DNA stands in bladder tumour cells. The support for intravesical installation for MMC comes from a meta-analysis by Sylvester et al. [7]. In this meta-analysis 7 randomized controlled trials were evaluated involving a total of

1476 patients with non-muscle invasive bladder cancer. This resulted in an absolute risk reduction of recurrences by 39%.

Table 1. The 2009 TNM classification of urinary bladder cancer

T - Primary tumour

TX Primary tumour cannot be assessed

T0 No evidence of primary tumour

Ta Non-invasive papillary carcinoma

Tis Carcinoma in situ: 'flat tumour'

T1 Tumour invades subepithelial connective tissue

T2 Tumour invades muscle

T2a Tumour invades superficial muscle (inner half)

T2b Tumour invades deep muscle (outer half)

T3 Tumour invades perivesical tissue:

T3a Microscopically

T3b Macroscopically (extravesical mass)

T4 Tumour invades any of the following: prostate, uterus, vagina, pelvic wall, abdominal wall

T4a Tumour invades prostate, uterus or vagina

T4b Tumour invades pelvic wall or abdominal wall

N - Lymph nodes

NX Regional lymph nodes cannot be assessed

N0 No regional lymph node metastasis

N1 Metastasis in a single lymph node in the true pelvis (hypogastric, obturator, external iliac, or presacral)

N2 Metastasis in multiple lymph nodes in the true pelvis (hypogastric, obturator, external iliac, or

presacral)

N3 Metastasis in common iliac lymph node(s)

M - Distant metastasis

MX Distant metastasis cannot be assessed

M0 No distant metastasis

M1 Distant metastasis

In patients with a diagnosis of Ta / T1 high grade disease patients undergo an early re-resection of the tumour as there is a significant risk of residual tumour [8]. The indications for early resection are after an incomplete initial TURBT; If there was no muscle in the specimen after initial resection, with exception of Ta G1 tumours/ primary CIS and in all T1 tumours and in all G3 tumours, except primary CIS.

There are several organizations that have proposed risk stratification for non-muscle invasive bladder cancer in the UK. The British Association of Urological Surgeons (BAUS) stratifies patients with non-muscle invasive bladder cancer into 3 risk groups (Low, Intermediate and High Risk). Low risk patients are those with pTa G1/G2 disease, the tumour is <3 cm and is solitary. Intermediate risk patients are those with pTa G1/G2 disease, tumour <3 cm and multiple or frequently recurring. The intermediate risk patients also consist of pT1 G2 and tumours < 3cm in diameter and solitary. High risk patients are those with pT1 G2 tumours which are > 3cm in diameter or multiple or chemoresistant. The pTa/pT1G3 and all high-grade tumours are categorized to be in the high risk group.

Patients with Ta/T1 G1/G2 (low) disease are managed with serial cystoscopies. In the event of patients developing non muscle invasive low grade (G1/G2) recurrences patients are normally given a course of intravesical MMC. This is given as 6 weekly installations of MMC. On the completion of these installations patients undergo serial cystoscopies.

In patients with a diagnosis of high-grade non muscle invasive Ta/T1 G3 tumours in the UK most patients undergo an early re-resection of the tumour. Once this disease has been confirmed to be Ta/T1G3 it is important to remember that the risk of progression in patients with Ta disease is 15%. T1G3 bladder cancer 30% of patients will never recur, 30% will undergo a deferred cystectomy and 30% will die from metastatic disease. Adjuvant immunotherapy with BCG is essential in these patients. In a study by Sylvester RJ et al. [9], the authors reviewed the data of 24 randomized controlled trials with a total of 4863 patients with non-muscle invasive high-risk bladder cancer. The absolute risk reduction of progression with BCG was 4% and the relative risk reduction of progression is 27%. Hence BCG was confirmed to reduced of progression. When T1G3 disease is association with CIS the risk of progression increases to 50-80%.

In patients with non-metastatic muscle invasive bladder cancer the treatment options include the role of Neo Adjuvant chemotherapy prior to radical cystectomy. Current literature indicates that overall survival benefit in patients undergoing neo adjuvant chemotherapy is 45% as against 50% at 5 years [10].

Conclusion

Haematuria is an important symptom of bladder cancer. In patients with visible haematuria and non-visible haematuria the diagnosis of bladder cancer can be seen in up to 20% of patients and 5% respectively. The prognosis of patients depends on the TNM stage and grade of the disease at diagnosis.

References

[1]   http://www.baus.org.uk/AboutBAUS/publications/haematuria-guidelines. 2008.

[2]   Vasdev N, Thorpe AC. Should the presence of a culture positive urinary tract infection exclude patients from rapid evaluation hematuria protocols? *Urol. Oncol.* 2013 Aug;31(6):909-13.

[3]   Khadra MH, Pickard RS, Charlton M, Powell PH, Neal DE. A prospective analysis of 1,930 patients with hematuria to evaluate current diagnostic practice. *Urol.* 2000 Feb;163(2):524-7.

[4]   Edwards TJ, Dickinson AJ, Natale S, Gosling J, McGrath JS. A prospective analysis of the diagnostic yield resulting from the attendance of 4020 patients at a protocol-driven haematuria clinic. *BJU Int.* 2006 Feb;97(2):301-5.

[5]   Jichlinski P., Leisinger H. (2005) Fluorescence cystoscopy in the management of bladder cancer: a help for the urologist! *Urol. Int.* 74: 97–101.

[6]   Sobin LH, Gospodariwicz M, Wittekind C (eds). TNM classification of malignant tumors. UICC International Union Against Cancer. 7th edn. Wiley-Blackwell, 2009 Dec; pp. 262-265.

[7]   Sylvester RJ1, Oosterlinck W, van der Meijden AP. A single immediate postoperative instillation of chemotherapy decreases the risk of recurrence in patients with stage Ta T1 bladder cancer: a meta-analysis of published results of randomized clinical trials. *J. Urol.* 2004 Jun;171(6 Pt 1):2186-90.

[8]   Vasdev N, Dominguez-Escrig J, Paez E, Johnson MI, Durkan GC, Thorpe AC. The impact of early re-resection in patients with pT1 high-grade non-muscle invasive bladder cancer. *Ecancermedicalscience.* 2012;6:269.

[9]   Sylvester RJ, van der MEIJDEN AP, Lamm DL. Intravesical bacillus Calmette-Guerin reduces the risk of progression in patients with superficial bladder cancer: a meta-analysis of the published results of randomized clinical trials. *J. Urol.* 2002 Nov;168(5):1964-70.

[10]   Vasdev N, Shaw M, Thorpe AC. Neoadjuvant chemotherapy in muscle invasive bladder cancer. *Curr. Urol.* 2011;5:57–61.

In: Hematuria
Editors: Nikhil Vasdev and G. Boustead

ISBN: 978-1-63463-073-3
© 2015 Nova Science Publishers, Inc.

Chapter 14

Barriers to the Early Diagnosis of Hematuria in Primary Care

James S. A. Green[1,2], Benjamin W. Lamb[1,3]
and Paula Allchorne[4]

[1]Department of Urology, Barts Health NHS Trust, London, UK
[2]Department of Health and Social Care, London Southbank University, London, UK
[3]Department of Surgery and Cancer, Imperial College London, London, UK
[4]Department of Urology, Guy's and St Thomas' NHS Foundation Trust, London, UK

Introduction/Background

In the UK there is a concern that patients with cancer present later with more advanced disease than their European counterparts. This delay in presentation appears to translate into lower survival rates compared to other countries [1, 2]. EUROCARE and CONCORD, two of the largest population based studies carried out on survivors of cancer, together with cancer statistics worldwide, appear to support this presumption [3, 4, 5, 6]. To address this issue there have been many initiatives over recent years to improve cancer survival by facilitating earlier diagnosis programs and shortening the time from diagnosis to definitive treatment. An example of this is the "two week wait (2WW) pathway". In this process any patient with suspected cancer is directed via a "fast track" pathway to be seen by a specialist within two weeks of referral by their general practitioner. Despite such proposals delays and barriers still occur.

Delays and Barriers in the Patient Pathway

Late presentation of cancer can be multi-factorial. But to resolve the contributing factors one can "map out" the patient pathway to unravel what may be causing the delay and at what point in the pathway this occurs. On reviewing the haematuria pathway there are multiple areas that can contribute to a delay in the patient's diagnosis (see Figure 1 below). In this chapter we will discuss factors affecting late presentation to the primary care practitioner (patient delay) and late referral by primary care practitioner (GP) to secondary care (GP delay and primary care system delay). In the following chapter we will discuss examples of systems delay in the primary care/secondary care interface, in the first secondary care visit and in diagnostic tests being carried out in secondary care (diagnostic delay) and subsequent potential barriers to definitive treatment [7].

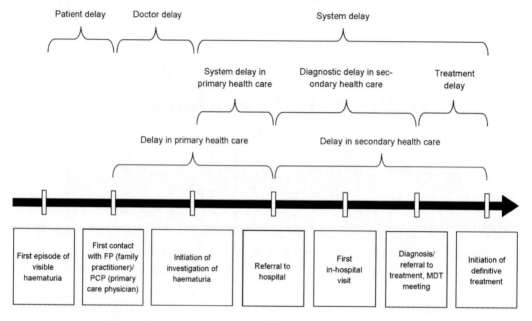

Figure 1. Categorisation of delay in a patient's haematuria pathway from onset of symptoms to definitive treatment.

Patient Factors

Patients' reactions to symptoms are complex. They are based on a multitude of factors ranging from the level of education and their past experiences to their current support structures. Whilst one patient may see an episode of painless visible haematuria (VH), that clears after a few days, as 'nothing to worry about' another will rush to the emergency department (ED) in a state of panic, and there is a whole continuum in between. Most clinicians dealing with bladder and renal cancer are often surprised when a patient seems relatively untroubled by a symptom as dramatic as visible painless haematuria and equally that patients with haematuria have little comprehension that bladder or renal cancer can present in this way. Unfortunately previous research demonstrates that public awareness of common cancers and their presenting symptoms is poor [9, 10]. Awareness is especially low among male, younger, and lower socio-economic status (SES) or ethnic minority patients. [11]. It is therefore not surprising that patients who may have bladder cancer or renal cancer presenting with haematuria are unaware of the significance of such symptoms.

In order to address the problem of lack of awareness of symptoms of cancer in the UK, in 2008 the National Awareness and Early Diagnosis Initiative (NAEDI) was formed [112]. NAEDI's key aim was to support projects and initiatives designed to promote the importance of earlier cancer diagnosis. The following year a novel report suggested that a combination of public education about symptoms, empowerment to seek medical advice, and support at primary care level could enhance early presentation and improve cancer outcomes [11]. To this end in 2011 NAEDI co-ordinated a national campaign 'Be Clear on Cancer' to raise public awareness of the signs and symptoms of cancer and to encourage people to seek advice from their GPs more promptly in order5 to improve early diagnosis. This public health initiative has been promoted through the media, with a targeted audience of men and women over the age of 50 of lower socio-economic backgrounds that may otherwise delay going to their GP for advice [13, 14]. So far the campaign has raised awareness of the signs and symptoms of bowel, lung and breast cancer, specifically targeting cancer groups that currently have inequalities in early diagnosis and treatment. Bladder and Renal Cancer patients are included in this category so in late 2013 it was the turn of 'visible haematuria' to take centre stage under the strap line of 'Blood in your Pee?'. To make this as successful as possible detailed research was undertaken to give it the most impact. Unsurprisingly the findings at the pilot sites for the project underlined a low level of public awareness. Knowledge of visible haematuria (VH) as a sign of potential malignancy was as low as 41% initially but increased to 65% following the educational campaign via television, radio and other advertisements. A second important finding from the pilot was that if the visible haematuria resolved, fairly quickly, it reassured people into thinking that the symptom was less important, with men being less likely to seek medical advice than women. This lead the campaign team to add the words, "even if it's just the once" to reiterate the important of this point [15].

There may also be other gender differences in haematuria and its initial recognition as a cancer symptom. Women may have more difficulty noticing haematuria in the first place. Not everybody inspects their urine each and every time before flushing the lavatory and it is not uncommon when questioned for women to say, "I never look at my pee" [16]. This may be a reason why some women have later presentation or tumours with worse prognosis than men. It is amusing to think that a potential improvement from the "Be clear on cancer" campaigns for bowel and bladder cancer may be as simple as more people inspecting the contents of their toilet bowl, but if that leads to earlier recognition of symptoms and treatment of serious cancers the campaign will have been a success.

Once a patient has noticed the haematuria, and realised that the symptom is significant, one would hope they would seek medical advice, but unfortunately some do not. There are known barriers to seeking help. The most common are difficulty making an appointment, worry about wasting the doctor's time and worry about what would be found, with emotional barriers being more prominent in lower SES groups and practical barriers (e.g., too busy) more prominent in higher SES groups [11] . In this regard much more work needs to be done on why patients with obvious symptoms delay in seeking medical advice and overcoming these issues.

In the important step of seeking medical advice, in the UK, there are two main choices that are available. The first is to seek advice from their local community based NHS primary care practitioner (general practitioner, GP or family physician, FP). The second is to choose to attend the emergency department (ED) if concerned about urgency or the severity of haematuria (see next chapter).

Primary Healthcare Factors

Primary Care is usually the first contact patients have with the health system regarding a problem that may be an indication of cancer. In countries like the UK and Denmark GPs are the gatekeepers who initiate the referral to secondary care. It is evident that patients need to present early to their GPs with potential symptoms, but just as importantly, GPs need to react to the symptom correctly. While many GPs realise the importance of painless visible haematuria as a symptom for urological malignancy, lesser degrees of haematuria (microscopic, invisible or nonvisible), and those accompanied by pain can lead to a diagnostic and referral conundrum for primary care physicians. This may be surprising to secondary care oncologists who deal with cancer on a daily basis but they have to remember that for primary care physicians benign disease is a far commoner explanation for most symptoms and this may skew their viewpoint.

An average GP will only see 8 or 9 new cases of cancer a year but several hundred may go to see their GP each year with symptoms that could potentially be due to cancer [17] To put this in clearer perspective, typically each year a GP will see only one new case each of breast, lung, prostate and colorectal cancer. They may only see some of the rarer cancers such as testicular about once every 20 years and a patient with a rare cancer once in their working lives [18]. A GP with a larger list size of 2000 people would expect to see approximately 3 new urological tumours in a year; Prostate 1- 2 cases (or possibly 3), Bladder 1, Renal 0.3, Testis, 0.1, Penis 0.02 [19].

Table 1. Number of all cancer types experienced by GPs related to population [16]

	Individual GP	Group practice	Primary Care Trust
Population	1,600	10,000	167,000
New cancer cases per annum	7-8	50	750
Patients with a cancer diagnosis	20-40	200	3,500
Deaths from cancer per annum	4	25	420
Home deaths from cancer	1	6	100

Most GP will make 25 2WW referrals a year for symptoms suspicious of cancer, which is only one per fortnight. Interestingly, there is a 3 fold variation between practitioners in two week wait referral rates (ranging from 900-2950 per 100,000 patients with an average of 1900) . Unravelling the factors that prompt these differing rates of cancer referral has proved to be very difficult. In one well conducted study no obvious GP characteristics stood out to explain this. Seniority, practice organization, list size, participation in continuing medical education, job satisfaction and level of burnout were not significantly associated with doctor delay in referral. Patients of female GPs more often had a short patient delay than patients of male GPs (OR 0.44, 95% confidence interval (95% CI) 0.28 to 0.71). Interestingly patients whose GPs provided many services (OR 0.66, 95% CI 0.44 to 0.95) and patients attending GPs with little former knowledge of their patients (OR 0.68, 95% CI 0.47 to 0.99) more often experienced a short system delay than patients attending GPs with less activity and more knowledge of their patients [20].

With regards urological cancers that present with haematuria, a man dying from bladder cancer is as rare as someone dying from pancreatic cancer. While a woman dying of renal cancer is rarer than a man dying of melanoma. As a GP will rarely see a patient with either bladder cancer or renal cancer it may not be upper most in their mind when they see a patient with haematuria and they may feel the need to exclude infection in women first when in fact recurrent UTI and haematuria can be exactly how bladder cancer may present. GPs who see relatively few cases of urological cancer may have difficulty identifying those at highest risk. In order to help GPs with this difficulty very clear guidelines on cancer symptoms were issued in 2001 by The National Institute for Health and Clinical Excellence (NICE), 'Referral guidelines for suspected cancer' aiming to ensure the prompt referral of a patient with possible signs or symptoms of cancer by the GP to secondary care [21].

Two studies have shown shortcomings in the timeliness of primary care referrals for urological cancer. A robust qualitative study in 2012 showed that GPs often diagnosed women with visible haematuria as suffering from urinary tract infections, despite being painless in nature, which delayed referral to secondary care for weeks or months. This led to some patients, desperate for access to a specialist opinion, to attend the emergency department [16]. Such findings have been echoed by a prospective national UK audit, which reviewed GP referral practices between 2009 and 2010. In 920 cases of bladder cancer and 398 of renal cancer the researchers identified poor practice in the timeliness of referrals of women with urological cancers. 27% (95% CI 21% to 33%) of women compared with 11% (9% to 14%) of men required three or more pre-referral consultations for bladder cancer (p<0.001); and 30% (22% to 39%) vs 18% (13% to 25%) for renal cancer (p=0.025). Women also had a greater number of days from presentation to referral. In multivariate analysis (adjusting for age, haematuria status and use of primary care-led investigations), being a woman was independently associated with higher odds of three or more pre-referral consultations for bladder cancer (OR=3.29 (2.06 to 5.25), p<0.001); and for renal cancer (OR=1.90 (1.06 to 3.42), p=0.031). Each year in the UK, approximately 700 women with either bladder or renal cancer experience a delayed diagnosis because of their gender, of whom more than a quarter (28%) present with haematuria. The researchers identified a need to both reinforce existing guidelines on haematuria investigation and develop new diagnostic decision aids and tests for patients who present with haematuria [22].

The "Blood in your Pee" advertising campaign appears to have empowered patient to take more control of their medical care to demand a referral to a haematuria clinic to investigate their symptoms further. This was evident in the pilot studies as 27% of people surveyed stated that they would seek a same day GP appointment if bladder habits changed after the campaign compared to 18% prior [23].

Conclusion

The main solution to overcome the barriers to care described above has its roots in health education. Specifically, the importance of recognising haematuria as a potential symptom for cancer and the need to refer on to the correct team in shortest time and most direct route possible. In the next chapter we will continue look at the haematuria pathway but concentrate on the access to and use of resources needed to diagnose and treat patients in order to improve outcomes and the barriers that can exist in these areas.

References

[1]   Ferlay, J., Shin, H.R., Bray, F., Forman, D., Mathers, C., Parkin, D.M. GLOBOCAN 2008 V1.2.Cancer Incidence and Mortality Worldwide: IARC Cancer Base No.10 (2010). Lyon, France: International Agency for Research on Cancer, WHO.

[2]   Cancer Research UK. Bladder Cancer Mortality Statistics. London: *Cancer Research UK*. 2012.

[3]   Verdecchia, A., Francisci, S., Brenner, H., Gatta, G., Micheli, A., Mangone, L., Kunkler, I. Recent cancer survival in Europe: a 2000-02 period analysis of EUROCARE-4 data. *The Lancet Oncology*. 2007. 8(9): 784-796.

[4]   Coleman, M., Quaresma, M., Berrino, F., et al. Cancer survival in five continents: a worldwide population-based study (CONCORD). *The Lancet Oncology*. 2008. 9(8): 730-756.

[5]   Berrino, F., De Angelis, R., Sant, M., et al. Survival for eight major cancers and all cancers combined for European adults diagnosed in 1995-99: results of the EUROCARE-4 study. *Lancet Oncology*. 2007. 8(9): 773-83.

[6]   Cancer Research UK. Worldwide Cancer Statistics. London: Cancer Research UK. 2012.

[7]   Foot, C., Harrison, T. How to improve cancer survival: Explaining England's relatively poor rates. London: King's Fund. 2011.

[8]   Olesen F, Hansen RP, Vedsted P. Delay in diagnosis: the experience in Denmark. *Br. J. Cancer*. 2009 Dec 3;101 Suppl 2:S5-8. doi: 10.1038/sj.bjc.6605383.

[9]   Brunswick, N., Wardle, J., Jarvis, M.J. Public awareness of warning signs for cancer in Britain. *Cancer Causes Control*. 2001 12: 33–37.

[10]   Stubbings, S., Robb, K., Waller, J., Ramirez, A., Austoker, J., Macleod, U., Hiom, S., Wardle, J. Development of a measurement tool to assess public awareness of cancer. *British Journal of Cancer*. 2009 101 (Suppl 2): S13–S17.

[11]   Robb K et al. Public awareness of cancer in Britain: a population-based survey of adults, Development of a measurement tool to assess public awareness of cancer, *British Journal of Cancer*. 2009 101, S18-S23.

[12]   National Awareness and Early Diagnosis Initiative. Available at: http://www.cancerresearchuk.org/cancer-info/spotcancerearly/naedi/AboutNAEDI/. Last accessed 10th April 2014.

[13]   Macleod, U., Mitchell, E.D., Burgess, C., Macdonald, S., Ramirez, A.J. Risk factors for delayed presentation and referral of symptomatic cancer: evidence for common cancers. *British Journal of Cancer*. 2009 101: S92-S101.

[14]   Department of Health. Evaluation of the bowel cancer awareness pilot. London: Stationary Office. 2012

[15]   NHS. Blood in Pee campaign fact sheet. Available at: http://www.cancerresearchuk.org/prod_consump/groups/cr_common/@nre/@hea/docu ments/image/cr_111044.pdf. Last accessed 10th April 2014.

[16] Allchorne P. Executive MBA in Health Service Management; Dissertation. Management Solutions to the barriers of early presentation to Bladder Cancer. Greenwich School of Management. University of Plymouth..

[17] Cancer Plan 2000. Department of Health. (2001 & 2003). *The Cancer Plan*. London: Stationary Office.

[18] Department of Health. Cancer Reform Strategy. London: Stationary Office. (2007).

[19] National Cancer Registry. Available from: http://www.ukacr.org/registration-organisation. Last accessed 10th April 2014.

[20] Hansen RP, Vedsted P, Sokolowski I, Søndergaard J, Olesen F. General practitioner characteristics and delay in cancer diagnosis. a population-based cohort study. *BMC Family Practice* 2011, 12:100

[21] National Institute for Health and Care Excellence. Referral guidelines for suspected cancer (CG27). Issued: June 2005 (last modified: April 2011). Available from: http://publications.nice.org.uk/referral-guidelines-for-suspected-cancer-cg27.   Last accessed 10th April 2014.

[22] Lyratzopoulos G, Abel GA, McPhail S, Neal RD, Rubin GP. Gender inequalities in the promptness of diagnosis of bladder and renal cancer after symptomatic presentation: evidence from secondary analysis of an English primary care audit survey. *BMJ Open* 2013;3:e002861

[23] Elliss-Brookes L, McPhail S, Ives A, Greenslade M, Shelton J, Hiom S, Richards M. Routes to diagnosis for cancer - determining the patient journey using multiple routine data sets. *Br. J. Cancer*. 2012 Oct 9;107(8):1220-6.

In: Hematuria
Editors: Nikhil Vasdev and G. Boustead

ISBN: 978-1-63463-073-3
© 2015 Nova Science Publishers, Inc.

Chapter 15

Inflammatory Causes of Hematuria

Prabhjot Singh, M.S., M.Ch.*, Siddharth Yadav, M.S.†
and Prem Nath Dogra, M.S., M.Ch.#
Department of Urology, All India institute of Medical Sciences,
New Delhi, India

Introduction

Hematuria is defined as presence of blood in the urine. It can be classified into visible (macroscopic) or nonvisible (microscopic). Asymptomatic nonvisible hematuria is present in 2.4- 31.1% of healthy men screened by microscopy and dipstick examination, with still higher rates amongst men over 60 years of age and in current or past smokers [1-6, 8-10]. With one episode of asymptomatic non visible hematuria chances of having significant urinary disease range from 0-56% [7] and chances of finding urologic malignancy ranges from 0-25.8% with overall malignancy rates of 2.6% [1-6, 8-10]. Thus every episode of hematuria should be thoroughly evaluated. The common causes of nonvisible hematuria are benign prostatic hyperplasia, infection and urinary calculi and that of visible hematuria include urinary bladder or upper tract malignancy. In a study of 110 patients with hematuria by Carter et al, malignancy was found in 22%. The common sites of primary cancer were bladder (9%), kidneys (6%), and prostate (6%). The common benign conditions causing hematuria were benign prostatic hypertrophy (19%), infection (26%), and stone disease (13.6%). [11]

* E-mail: drprabhjotsingh@gmail.com.
† E-mail: siddhi666@ymail.com.
# E-mail: premnathdogra@gmail.com.

Evaluation

Hematuria is usually an alarming symptom for the patient and proper history can be valuable in localizing the cause. Blood in the initial portion of urine usually arises from urethra that, in the terminal portion of urine, arises from bladder neck or posterior urethra and total hematuria results from causes above the bladder neck that is bladder, ureter or kidneys. Symptomatic hematuria usually results from benign causes. Hematuria with colicky pain is caused by stone disease and that associated with dysuria is caused by urinary tract infection or carcinoma in situ. Painless visible hematuria is indicator of urothelial or renal malignancy. History of weight loss, arthralgias, systemic illness or drug intake especially antiplatelet or anticoagulant therapy or any family history of hematuria or hearing loss and travel to Middle Eastern countries should be elicited. Presence of petechiae, arthritis, or rash on general examination suggests coagulopathy, or vasculitis as the cause. Local examination of genitalia and digital rectal examination identify benign and malignant urethral and prostatic diseases.

Dipstick analysis is usually the first test to indentify hematuria in cases suspicious to naked eye. It is semi quantitative and detects heame thus cannot distinguish between hematuria, hemoglobinuria and myoglobinuria. If dipstick examination is positive microscopic examination of urine is recommended to confirm the diagnosis [12]. Presence of 3 or more RBC/HPF on microscopic examination of urine is regarded as microscopic hematuria. Presence of red blood cell casts or dysmorphic red blood cells (especially acanthocytes – erythrocytes with ring form) in urine signifies hematuria of glomerular origin. Hematuria along with proteinuria more than 0.5grams/day, hypertension or estimated GFR <60ml/min warrants further nephrology evaluation for glomerular or tubular diseases. Presence of pus cells or bacteria along with red blood cells indicates urinary tract infection.

Single episode of visible hematuria, symptomatic non visible hematuria or isolated hematuria (hematuria without proteinuria) needs further urologic evaluation. Patients on anticoagulants should also be evaluated as 25% of them may have underlying abnormality [13]. Multidetector computed tomography (MDCT) is the current imaging investigation of choice. It should include a preenhancement phase to detect baseline density of tissues and high or variable density such as calculi, hematoma and fat containing structure, an arterial phase to identify neoplastic and inflamatory neovascularity, a corticomedullary phase to evaluate renal parenchyma and an excretory phase to detect abnormalities of collecting system. Sensitivity and specificity of MDCT is above 90% (sensitivity- 96% specificity 99%) [14]. The risk of contrast induced nephropathy, allergic reaction and radiation associated with CT scans are well known and if these conditions preclude CT, magnetic resonance urography is (MRU) an acceptable alternative. MRU has high sensitivity and specificity (more than 90%) in imaging renal parenchyma and identifying obstruction. However the role of MRU in identifying collecting system lesions is not yet established. If imaging of collecting system is deemed necessary, combining MRI with retrograde pyelogram (RGP) is advisable. RGP, although invasive, is a safe way to evaluate entire upper tracts for filling defects, obstruction and irregularity. If condition preclude both contrast enhanced computed tomography (CECT) and magnetic resonance imaging (MRI) then non contrast CT with RGP is an option. Ultrasonography, which is usually the first line investigation, is usually not diagnostic and irrespective of the result of scan, further evaluation is usually required. It is good modality for imaging renal lesions (sensitivity 100%) but misses many transitional cell carcinomas specially in upper urinary tracts (sensitivity 50%) [15]. Intravenous urography (IVU) was earlier the imaging modality of choice for evaluation of hematuria with sensitivity of 60% and specificity of 90% [16] but with the advent of CT urogram, it is no longer recommended. Combination of IVU and USG is less acceptable alternative to CTU as these techniques do not provide diagnostic certainity.

Table. Inflammatory Causes of Hematuria

Urinary tract infection
Cystitis
Prostatitis
Pyelonephritis
Urethritis
Stone disease
Tuberculosis
Schistosomiasis
Stricture urethra

Cystoscopy is recommended in patients older than 35yr of age or in those with risk factors for urinary tract malignancy like tobacco exposure, chemical exposure or irritative voiding symptoms [12]. All patients with hematuria and non diagnostic imaging who fulfill above criteria should undergo cystoscopy to identify the origin of hematuria.

Urinary Tract Infection (UTI)

Inflammation anywhere in urinary tract may result in hematuria. Urinary tract infections are more common in women, older age groups and in patients with indwelling catheter. Cystitis causes transient symptomatic non visible hematuria that subsides with treatment. It is most commonly caused by Escherichia Coli (E.coli). In sexually active females Staphylococcus saprophyticus is the second most common organism after E. coli. These patients present with dysuria, frequency and/or urgency with/without suprapubic pain and foul smelling urine. Dipstick test positive for nitrite and leukocyte esterase is a quick and easy test but identifying bacteriuria, pyuria and hematuria on microscopic examinations makes diagnosis of cystitis. Definitive diagnosis can be made on urine culture and presence of 100 cfu/ml of bacteria is diagnostic of cystitis in a symptomatic patient. Three day course of cotrimoxazole in females and 7 days course in men is generally acceptable treatment and hematuria should resolve with resolution of infection. Recurrent hematuria or recurrent UTI warrants further evaluation.

Pyelonephritis is inflammation of kidney and renal pelvis caused by ascent of bacteria from urinary bladder. Classic presentation is fever with chills and rigor and flank pain. Urine analysis shows hematuria, bacteriuria, and pyuria with presence of granular or leucocyte casts. Bacteria are demonstrable within the casts after staining with KOVA or toluidine blue. Urine cultures are positive only in 20% of the patients with pyelonephritis with E. coli being the commonest organism isolated. Fourteen day course of antibiotics is recommended with post treatment urine cultures to document eradication because of 10-30% risk of relapse following treatment.

Prostatitis is the most common urologic diagnosis in men less than 50 yrs of age and is commonly caused by E. coli. In patients who present with sepsis, suprapubic and perineal pain and lower urinary tract symptoms acute bacterial prostatitis should be suspected. Urinary culture is enough to make the diagnosis and prostatic massage is contraindicated. In contrast, chronic bacterial prostatitis presents as recurrent UTI due to focal areas of uropathogenic organism residing in the prostate gland. 10 fold increase in bacterial counts after prostatic massage clinches the diagnosis of chronic bacterial prostatitis. Antibiotic therapy for 2-4 weeks is usually required to eliminate infection.

Urethral inflammation is most often caused by bacteria, commonly Neisseria gonorrhea and Chlamydia trachomatis. Patients usually present with dysuria and urethral discharge. Presence of mucopurulent discharge, >5 WBC / HPF in urethral secretions, >10 WBC/HPF in initial voided urine specimen or leukocyte esterase test positive in initial voided urine specimen makes the diagnosis of urethritis. Identification of diplococcus in gram stain of urethral secretions is diagnostic for gonococcal urethritis. Nucleic acid amplification test (NAAT) on initial voided urine specimen accurately detects gonococcal and chlamydial urethritis. Dual therapy is recommended because the patients are usually coinfected and Cefixime 400mg single dose with Azithromycin 1gm single dose is the recommended regimen.

Tuberculosis

Genitourinary tuberculosis is second most common type of extra pulmonary tuberculosis and accounts for 30-40% of all extra pulmonary cases [17]. Hematogenous spread of bacilli, in 20-25% of patients with pulmonary tuberculosis, results in genitourinary tuberculosis. Kidneys, epididymis, prostate and fallopian tubes are the primary landing sites of bacilli and other organs are affected either by direct, endoluminal or lymphatic spread. Kidneys are the most commonly affected organs and cortex is favored over medulla due to greater blood supply and higher oxygen tension. Infection leads to tubercle formation in renal parenchyma with central caseation, which later coalesce to form large abscesses. As the disease progresses caseation spreads to tubules and renal medulla. Renal papillary involvement results in sloughing and caseous material enters the collecting system leading to pyuria and hematuria. Healing occurs with fibrosis causing infundibular stenosis or pelviureteric junction scarring leading to hydronephrosis [18].

Ureteric involvement results from endoluminal passage of caseous material from the kidneys and is characterized by tubercle formation on the mucosa. Ureterovesical junction is the most commonly involved segment that later, as disease progresses, gets fibrosed leading to stricture formation and obstruction [19]. Bladder is resistant to tubercle bacilli and is involved late in course of disease due to direct extension from the kidneys. Area near the ureteric orifice and trigone is most commonly affected with tubercle formation. These may coalesce to form tuberculous ulcer with undermined margins and worm eaten ragged edges.

Tubercular epididymitis starts at globus minor because of its high vascularity and then spreads to rest of epididymis. Testes may be involved by direct extension secondary to epididymal disease in advanced cases. Prostate and seminal vesicle are rarely involved. Genitourinary tuberculosis is more common in males with storage lower urinary tract symptoms as the usual presentation. Hematuria can be present in one third of cases [20] and constitutional symptoms occur in less than 20% of cases [21]. Thickened nodular non-tender epididymis is most common finding on examination [20].

Urine microscopy typically shows sterile pyuria which can be the only finding in 25% of cases and 13% patients present with gross or microscopic hematuria only [22]. Urine for Ziehl Neelsen staining is often negative and 3-5 early morning samples cultured soon after collection is usually required to make the diagnosis. Urinary cultures have sensitivity in range of 80-90% and specificity of 100% [23]. Urine PCR for amplification of DNA and RNA of tubercle bacilli shows sensitivity of 87-95% and specificity of 92-99.8%. However these tests can amplify the nucleic acid of dead organism and thus can give false positive result and should be used only for diagnosis and not for follow up.

IVU is the most commonly performed radiologic investigation to diagnose genitourinary TB and hydrocalicosis, hydronephrosis and hydroureter are the most common findings. Moth eaten appearance of calyxes and irregularity of papilla are seen in early stages of disease and as the disease progresses there is distortion of collecting system or pelviureteric junction obstruction with hydronephrosis because of scarring. Computed tomography although less commonly used, is the most sensitive imaging modality and detects early lesions such as renal parenchymal abscesses and scars. Cystoscopy is rarely required, and there are no pathognomic findings. Biopsy of lesions is positive only in 18-45% of cases [24, 25] but it rules out malignancy.

Short course chemotherapy (Antitubercular therapy 6-9 months) is currently the management of choice with Directly Observed Therapy to ensure patient compliance. Surgery is reserved to either relieve obstruction or extirpative if the unit is nonfunctioning despite adequate drainage and medical management. Bladder augmentation may be required if capacity becomes less than 100ml.

Schistosomiasis

Schistosomiasis is parasitic infection caused by trematode Schistosoma. Out of S. japonicum, S. mansoni and S haematobium, S. haematobium resides in perivesical venous plexus resulting in urinary schistosomiasis and is endemic in countries of Middle East and African continent. Schistosomiasis results when cercariae – fork tailed larval stage of S. haematobium- present in fresh water, penetrates unbroken skin of human host. Adult worms migrate to venous plexus of urinary bladder and deposit their eggs into wall of urinary bladder. The terminally spined eggs of S hematobium pass through the urinary bladder wall causing intense inflammatory reaction and are excreted in urine.

Schistosomiasis results from granulomatous inflammatory response against the eggs [26]. During active infection, all stages of granuloma are simultaneously present which form large, bulky, hyperemic, inflammatory polyps projecting into lumen of bladder [27].

Hematuria is usually the first sign of schistosomiasis and occurs 10-12 weeks after the infection [28]. Hematuria, terminal dysuria, urgency, frequency and lower abdominal and perineal pain characterize established infection. In the later stages, inflammatory lesions are replaced by fibrosis and thickening of bladder wall occurs reducing the capacity of bladder and causing ureteric obstruction with hydroureter. Diagnosis of schistosomiasis is made by documenting terminally spined eggs in urinary sediment or stool samples. If eggs are not detected in urinary sediment, rectal or bladder biopsies can be attempted. USG may show non specific bladder wall thickening with polypoidal masses. IVU may reveal calcification in bladder or ureteral wall, hydroureter, hydrouretronephrosis, non-functioning kidney or vesicoureteric reflux.

Medical management with praziquantel is treatment of choice and surgical treatment is reserved for complications that do not respond. Most common elective surgery in patients with schistosomiasis is to relieve obstruction and severe bladder hemorrhage is commonest presentation needing urgent intervention.

Stone Disease

Ten to fifteen percent of general population is affected by urinary calculi [29, 30]. Calculi are more common in white obese men in fourth to sixth decade of life residing in hot arid regions. Patients usually are symptomatic and present with flank pain radiating from loin to groin depending on the location of stone. Urine analysis reveals pyuria and hematuria with or without bactiuria. Urinary tract calculi results in non visible hematuria and comprises of 6% of all the cases of hematuria [12]. Non Contrast spiral CT followed CT urogram is the imaging modality of choice. Management strategies depend on the site and burden of stone.

Urethral Stricture

Urethral stricture is fibrotic narrowing that extends into the corpus spongiosum causing spongiofibrosis due to deposition of collagen and elastin. It causes 1.4% of all cases of non visible hematuria. Most of inflammatory strictures are caused by indwelling catheters and gonococcal strictures, which were earlier the commonest cause, are seldom seen these days. Patients usually present with obstructive lower urinary tract symptoms with poor stream and straining. Long-standing stricture can be complicated by urinary retention, acute cystitis, prostatitis, epididymoorchitis, and periurethral abcess or urethrocutaneous fistula. Urine microscopic examination reveals pyuria and hematuria, bactiuria is occasionally seen. Management depends on location, length and tightness of stricture segment.

Conclusion

Visible hematuria is usually caused by malignancy. Every single episode of hematuria should be thoroughly evaluated and malignant causes should always be ruled out. Cystoscopy should be included in the work up of the hematuria when imaging modalities fail to identify a cause. Inflammatory causes need thorough evaluation and diagnosis followed by treatment of specific cause.

References

[1] Messing E. M., Young T. B., Hunt V. B., et al. The significance of asymptomatic micro hematuria in men 50 or more years old: findings of a home screening study using urinary dipsticks. *J. Urol.*, 1987: 137: 919.

[2] Messing E. M., Young T. B., Hunt V. B., et al. Urinary tract cancers found by homescreening with hematuria dipsticks in healthy men over 50 years of age. *Cancer,* 1989; 64: 2361.

[3] Messing E. M., Young T. B., Hunt V. B. et al. Home screening for hematuria: results of a multiclinic study. *J. Urol.,* 1992; 148: 289.

[4] Messing E. M., Young T. B., Hunt V. B., et al. Hematuria home screening: repeat testing results. *J. Urol.,* 1995; 154: 57.

[5] Britton J. P., Dowell A. C. and Whelan P. Dipstick haematuria and bladder cancer in men over 60: results of a community study. *BMJ,* 1989; 299: 1010.

[6] Britton J. P., Dowell A. C., Whelan P., et al. A community study of bladder cancer screening by the detection of occult urinary bleeding. *J. Urol.,* 1992; 148: 788.

[7] Grossfeld G. D., Litwin M. S., Wolf J. S., et al. Evaluation of asymptomatic microscopic hematuria in adults: the American Urological Association Best Practice Policy-Part I: definition, detection, prevalence, and etiology. *Urology,* 2001; 57:599–603.

[8] Emamian S. A., Nielsen M. B. and Pedersen J. F. Can dipstick screening for hematuria identify individuals with structural renal abnormalities? A sonographic evaluation. *Scand. J. Urol. Nephrol.,* 1996; 30: 25.

[9] Haug K., Bakke A., Daae L. N., et al: Screening for hematuria, glucosuria and proteinuria in people aged 55-64. Technical, clinical and cost-benefit experience from a pilot study. *Scand. J. Prim. Health Care,* 1985; 3: 31.

[10] Hedelin H., Jonsson K., Salomonsson K. et al: Screening for bladder tumours in men aged 60-70 years with a bladder tumour marker (UBC) and dipstick-detected haematuria using both white-light and fluorescence cystoscopy. *Scand. J. Urol. Nephrol.,* 2006; 40: 26.

[11] Carter W. C., Rous S. N. Gross hematuria in 110 adult urologic hospital patients. *Urology,* 1981; 18:342–344.

[12] Davis R., Jones J. S., Barocas D. A., et al. Diagnosis, evaluation and follow-up of asymptomatic microhematuria (AMH) in adults: AUA guideline. *J. Urol.,* 2012; 188: 2473-81.

[13] Van Savage J. G., Fried F. A. Anticoagulant associated hematuria: a prospective study. *J. Urol.,* 1995;153:1594-6.

[14] Chlapoutakis K., Theocharopoulos N., Yarmenitis S., et al: Performance of computed tomographic urography in diagnosis of upper urinary tract urothelial carcinoma, in patients presenting with hematuria: Systematic review and meta-analysis. *Eur. J. Radiol.,* 2010; 73: 334.

[15] Datta S. N., Allen G. M., Evans R., et al: Urinary tract ultrasonography in the evaluation of haematuria--a report of over 1,000 cases. *Ann. R. Coll. Surg. Engl.,* 2002; 84: 203.

[16] Gray Sears C. L., Ward J. F., Sears S. T., et al: Prospective comparison of computerized tomography and excretory urography in the initial evaluation of asymptomatic microhematuria. *J. Urol.*, 2002; 168: 2457.

[17] Eastwood J. B., Corbishley C. M., Grange J. M. Tuberculosis and the kidney. *J. Am. Soc. Nephrol.*, 2001 Jun.;12:1307-14.

[18] Medlar E. M. Cases of renal infection in pulmonary tuberculosis : Evidence of healed tuberculous lesions. *Am. J. Pathol.*, 1926 ;1:401-414.

[19] Shin K. Y., Park H. J., Lee J. J., et al. Role of endourologic management of tuberculous uretral strictures. *J. Endourol.*, 2002;16:755-8.

[20] Figueieredo A. A., Lucon A. M., Gomes C. M.,et al.Urogenital tuberculosis: patient classification in seven different groups according to clinical and radiological presentation. *Int. Braz. J. Urol.*, 2008;34:422-32.

[21] Simon H. B., Weinstein A. J., Pasternak M. S., et al. Genitourinary tuberculosis. Clinical features in a general hospital population. *Am. J. Med.,* 1977 ;63:410-20.

[22] Wise G. J., Shtenshlyuger A. An update on lower urinary tract tuberculosis. *Curr. Urol. Rep.*, 2008; 9: 305-13.

[23] Sorlozano A., Soria I., Roman J., Huertas P., et al. Comparative evaluation of three culture methods for the isolation of mycobacteria from clinical samples. *J. Microbiol. Biotechnol.*, 2009 ;19:1259-64.

[24] Wong S. H., Lau W. Y., Poon G. P., et al. The treatment of urinary tuberculosis. *J. Urol.*, 1984;131:297-301.

[25] Hemal A. K., Gupta N. P., Rajeev T. P., Kumar R., Dar L., Seth P. Polymerase chain reaction in clinically suspected genitourinary tuberculosis: comparison with intravenous urography, bladder biopsy, and urine acid fast bacilli culture. *Urology,* 2000; 56:570-4.

[26] Phillips S. M., Colley D. G. Immunologic aspects of host responses to schistosomiasis: resistance, immunopathology, and eosinophil involvement. *ProgAllergy,* 1978; 24: 49-182.

[27] Smith J. H., Kelada A. S., Khalil A., et al. Surgical pathology of schistosomal obstructive uropathy: a clinicopathologic correlation. *Am. J. Trop. Med. Hyg.,* 1977; 26: 96-103.

[28] Kehinde E. O., Anim J. T., Hira P. R. Parasites of urologic importance. *Urol. Int.,* 2008;81:1-13.

[29] Norlin A., Lindell B., Granberg P. O., Lindvall N. Urolithiasis. A study of its frequency. *Scand. J. Urol. Nephrol.*, 1976;10:150-3.

[30] Sierakowski R., Finlayson B., Landes R. R., et al. The frequency of urolithiasis in hospital discharge diagnosis in United States. *Invest. Urol.,* 1978;15:438-41.

In: Hematuria
Editors: Nikhil Vasdev and G. Boustead

ISBN: 978-1-63463-073-3
© 2015 Nova Science Publishers, Inc.

Chapter 16

Management of Haematuria in Patients with Prostate Cancer

Benjamin W. Lamb[1,2], Chi-Ying Li[1], Wei-Shen Tan[1,3] and James S. A. Green[1,4]

[1]Whipps Cross University Hospital,
Barts Health NHS Trust, London, UK
[2]Department of Surgery and Cancer, Imperial College London, UK
[3]Department of Urology, University College London, UK
[4]Department of Health and Social Care, Southbank
University, London, UK

Introduction

The prevalence of haematuria in the general population has been estimated to be 2.5%, of whom 13% are found to have a urological malignancy [1]. In our own institution, we found that 34% of patients who presented to the emergency department with visible haematuria had an underlying malignancy, and of the men 14% had prostate cancer [2]. Moreover, haematuria in the context of prostate cancer may arise as a result of the underlying condition, its treatment (e.g., radiotherapy), or an associated condition (e.g., BPH)

In this chapter we discuss the initial assessment and management of patients with haematuria, which will be sufficient to control the problem in the majority of patients. For rare cases where initial measures are not sufficient to stop the haematuria, we review the evidence for the use of additional physical, chemical and radiological measures which may become necessary.

Acute Assessment

Presentation

Haematuria can present with visible (macroscopic) or non-visible (microscopic / dipstick) haematuria. Patients with visible haematuria that does not require management as an inpatient and those with non-visible haematuria can usually be investigated on an outpatient basis, in line with guidance from the British Association of Urological Surgeons and the Renal Association, to exclude other urological malignancies [3].

Patients requiring admission to hospital include those with cardiovascular compromise or clot retention. Patients with prostate cancer can present with haematuria either as a result of the prostate cancer itself, as a complication of the treatment for their prostate cancer, or from causes unrelated to the prostate cancer. It is important to recognise that patients with prostate cancer can also develop other cancers of the urinary tract that can present with haematuria; so, it is important not to miss identifying other urological malignancies, while managing the haematuria.

History

A thorough history and examination should be carried out which may give some indication as to the origin of the haematuria [4]. The duration of haematuria should be ascertained.

Patients with visible haematuria are at risk of developing clot retention, therefore enquiring about the presence of clots, and the ability to void is important. Inability to void or the presence of large clots requires treatment by insertion of a large bore 3-way catheter and initiation of bladder washout to remove the clots, followed by bladder irrigation (see below). Pain associated with haematuria suggests urinary tract calculus. Lower urinary tract symptoms and fever suggest urinary tract infection (UTI), it is important to identify signs of sepsis and initiate appropriate management with early use of intravenous antimicrobials. Culture and sensitivity results from previous infections, if available, may help to direct the selection of an appropriate anti-microbial regimen.

History of recent urological instrumentation may suggest iatrogenic cause, or indicate pathology already under investigation as the likely cause of the visible haematuria. Further specific enquiries should be made in patients with a pre-existing diagnosis of prostate cancer, it is important to ask about; diagnosis, treatment received - including both previous and current therapy, disease status - including known metastatic disease and most recent Prostate Specific Antigen (PSA) level.

Any history of previous pelvic radiotherapy for prostate or other malignancy, which may increase the risk of developing haemorrhagic radiation cystitis, or bladder tumour, or potentially prevent patients from receiving further radiotherapy as treatment for their haematuria.

Previous medical history, especially of conditions that may increase a patient's risk of bleeding (e.g., coagulopathies), medication history (especially the use of any anticoagulant and the indication for this treatment) should be sought. Consideration should be given to the potential risks and benefits of omitting or reversing this treatment, this may require consultation with other specialist teams and further investigation with coagulation studies. An assessment should be made of exposure to risks factors for other urological malignancies [5]. Table 1 below summarises risk factors associated with other urological malignancies which may present with haematuria.

Table 1.

Site	Risk factors
Renal tumour	Smoking, obesity, hypertension, first degree relatives with history of Renal Cell Carcinoma, renal failure and dialysis.
Ureteric tumour	Smoking, occupational exposure to aromatic amines (benzidine and beta-naphthalene used in industries including dyes, textiles and rubber industries, however these have been banned since the 1960s in most industrialised countries) Aristolochic acid found in some Chinese Herbal Medicine and in Balkan nephropathy
Bladder tumour	Smoking (ex-smoker) Occupational exposure (as above) Pelvic radiotherapy (prostate cancer) Cyclophosphomide / Pioglitazone Schistosomiasis Long term urethral catheter

Examination

The most important features to identify as part of the physical examination include: cardiovascular status, the presence of a palpable bladder and signs of other urological malignancies. Cardiovascular compromise requires immediately resuscitation. The presence of a palpable bladder suggests acute or impending urinary retention and requires decompression with a 3-way urinary catheter as discussed previously. Signs of other urological malignancies include the presence of a palpable mass in the loin, or signs of metastatic disease such as cervical lymphadenopathy. Digital rectal examination should be carried out to assess the size of the prostate and to allow an assessment of the clinical stage of the prostatic malignancy.

Laboratory Tests

Mid-stream urine (MSU), if patient is able to void, should be collected and a urine dipstick test carried out. Absence of leucocyte and nitrite would significantly reduce the likelihood of a UTI, but does not completely exclude the diagnosis. Formal investigation with laboratory microscopy, culture and sensitivity should be requested. Previous urinary culture results can be very helpful, as patients with recurrent urinary infection in the context of prostate cancer, tend to develop UTI as a result of bacterial persistence due to underlying functional or anatomical abnormality of the urinary tract. Therefore, they tend to experience reinfection with the same organism, displaying similar antimicrobial sensitivities [5]. In the absence of current culture and sensitivity results, a pragmatic approach would be the use of previous positive MSU sensitivities to guide therapy, while the results of new investigations are awaited. Alternatively, if no MSU results are available, the UTI should be treated according to local antimicrobial policy.

Other laboratory tests which are helpful in the acute management of visible haematuria include; a Full Blood Count (FBC), Urea and Electrolyte (U&E) including estimated Glomerular Filtration rate (eGFR) and Group & Save of serum. Consideration should also be given to a coagulation screen in selected patients. FBC indicates the haemoglobin level, the presence of thrombocytopenia, or the presence of a raised white cell count as a marker of infection. U&E may demonstrate impaired renal function, and indicate whether this may be acute or chronic.

In patients with prostate cancer this may suggest urinary tract obstruction requiring decompression both at the bladder and bilateral ureteric levels. A recent PSA result may indicate disease status (in PSA secreting prostate cancers).

It is of some debate if a clotting profile should be a standard investigation in all patients with haematuria as it is a poor screening tool for new bleeding diatheses. A pragmatic approach should be adopted: in patients with known clotting disorder, bleeding diathesis, or underlying disease process which may affect clotting (e.g., liver dysfunction) and in those taking anticoagulants, a clotting profile should be checked. In patients with a significant amount of haematuria, a transfusion sample for blood (Group and Save) should be performed and in those with haemodynamic compromise, urgent cross-matching should be requested.

Radiology

In prostate cancer patients with visible haematuria, radiological investigation has two main roles. Firstly, radiological investigation is necessary to exclude other malignancies of the urinary tract, and secondly, to investigate and treat an identifiable bleeding point. To investigate suspected urinary tract malignancy, CT IVU is the investigation of choice. However, the use of radiological contrast has some important contraindications – in particular a known allergy to contrast media. The risk of developing contrast induced acute kidney injury must also be considered.

For patients with haematuria refractory to conservative methods, angiography with or without embolisation can be considered (see below). In those with significant renal impairment or contraindication to receiving contrast, ultrasound KUB or CT KUB can be considered. However, it must be acknowledged that if ultrasound is the solitary imaging modality used to identify suspected urinary tract malignancy, a small proportion of urothelial tumours may be missed [1].

Resuscitation

In patients with haemodynamic compromise, immediate resuscitation must be initiated. The goals of resuscitation focus on systematically managing impairment to airway, breathing and circulation. Circulatory support involves large bore intravenous access, sending blood for cross matching, appropriate fluid volume replacement – or blood transfusion, correction of any coagulopathy and urinary drainage with urine output monitoring.

Acute Management of Haematuria

Bladder Washout and Irrigation (Box 1)

The initial management of patients with gross haematuria with clots involves the insertion of a large calibre three way Foley catheter (ideally at least 22Fr) [6]. Bladder washout with a 50ml bladder syringe and prophylactic antibiotic (often gentamycin) cover should be performed using aseptic technique until the bladder is free of clots to prevent the catheter from becoming blocked. In the hands of trained personnel, the Foley catheter balloon can be deflated and bladder wash out be performed to evacuate clots near the bladder neck.

Box 1.

Technique for bladder washout and commencement of irrigation fluid
Equipment needed:
- 3 way catheter (ideally 22Fr)
- Local anaesthetic lubrication jelly
- Y connector
- 50ml bladder syringe
- Sterile gloves 2X
- Catheter pack
- Personal protective equipment
- 2X 2l bottles of 0.9% saline

Technique for patients presenting initially with haematuria and clots:
1) Explain to the patient about the procedure
2) Insert 3 way catheter into bladder using standard aseptic technique
3) Ensure urine is draining from catheter prior to commencing washout
4) Inject 50ml of 0.9% NaCl into bladder (forcefully if the patient has had no previous bladder tumour resection to break up large clots) and aspirate fluid back and discard aspirated fluid
5) Repeat procedure till no further clots are seen.
6) Fill the folly catheter balloon with 20ml of water and pull the cather back to ensure the balloon is the bladder neck
7) Connect the Y connector after it has been primed with 0.9% NaCl and start irrigation fluid
8) The speed of irrigation fluid should be dependent on how dark the haematuria of the patient is

Technique for patients presenting with clot obstruction despite on bladder irrigation:
1) Obtain a history and examine the patient for the presence of suprapubic pain, vasovagal symptoms, bypassing around catheter, the absence of irrigation fluid flowing into bladder or the absence of urine/ irrigation fluid output
2) Attempt to aspirate clots with a 50ml bladder syringe
3) If aspiration fails, use approximately 50 ml of 0.9% NaCl and inject it into the bladder with the aim to dislodge the blood clot and the bladder syringe aspirated
4) If aspiration is difficult, consider deflating the balloon of the catheter to try dislodge the clot.
5) Failing which, the catheter should be changed (consider a larger calibre catheter)
6) Continue to perform step 3 till there are no further clots and haematuria is rosé
7) If bleeding is an issue inflate the balloon of the catheter to 30ml and consider 20 minutes of traction of the catheter.
8) Irrigation fluid should be run as fast as possible to prevent recurrent clot formation
9) If clots are still persistent or the patient is hemodynamically unstable, consider GA cystoscopy and bladder washout with Ellik evacuator

---

In patients with no recent history of bladder tumour resection, a rigorous bladder wash-out can help break up large clots to aid successful clot evacuation. After all clots have been evacuated, bladder irrigation should be commenced to prevent the formation of any further clots. Care must be taken to ensure that the bladder is as empty as possible before instilling further fluid in to the bladder in order not to over distend an already full bladder, risking bladder perforation.

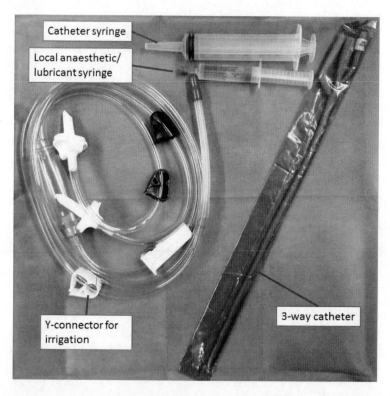

Figure 1. Apparatus for performing bladder washout and irrigation. Displayed are Y-connector, bladder syringe, local anaesthetic lubricant gel, three way catheter.

0.9% sodium chloride (NaCl) is the irrigation fluid of choice. A Y-connector with two bottles of irrigation fluid should be used to maintain continuity of irrigation to prevent clot formation. Water should not be used to prevent dilution hypernatremia and fluid overload [7] (Figure 1).

In the event that a patient develops a palpable bladder, suprapubic pain, fluid leaking around the catheter (bypassing) or vasovagal symptoms, catheter lumen obstruction secondary to blood clot needs to be rule out. The patient should be examined and their medical notes reviewed. Inspect the catheter drainage bag to determine the catheter is still draining. If this is not the case, irrigation fluid should be stopped. A 50ml bladder syringe should be used to aspirate the clot. If this fails, a 0.9% NaCl filled 50ml bladder syringe should be used to forcefully inject fluid into the bladder with the aim to dislodge the clot at the eye of the catheter. The bladder syringe is then used to aspirate from the outlet channel to try to evacuate the clot. This process is repeated until no further clot is aspirated and the haematuria is rosé in colour. If fluid is easily injected into the bladder but there is resistance aspirating fluid, a clot might be adhering to the eye of the catheter. Occasionally, deflating the balloon might dislodge the clot and aid a successful bladder washout. Always remember to re-inflate the balloon after. If deflating the catheter balloon fails to help, the catheter should be changed, possibly to a larger calibre catheter. Irrigation fluid should be run as fast as possible to prevent the risk of repeated clot retention. If bleeding is an issue, consider inflating the catheter balloon to 30ml of water to tamponade the bleeding. Persistent bleeding might require traction for 20 minutes to stop bleeding. Several studies have suggested instillation of hydrogen peroxide or chymotrypsin into the bladder via Foley catheter to help break up organised clots but these studies were based on small case series [8,9] (Figure 2).

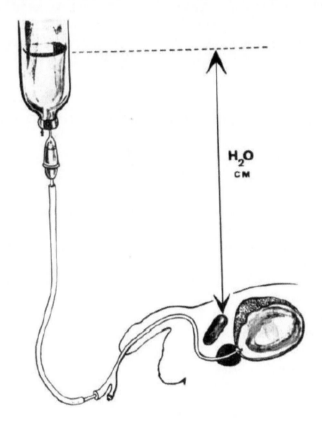

Figure 2. Original image from Helmstien's description of Hydrodistension in 1972.

Cystoscopy and Bladder Washout

If patients continue to develop repeated catheter obstruction despite irrigation fluid and repeated bladder washout or if the patient is hemodynamically unstable, a general anaesthetic (GA) cystoscopy with washout should be considered. Organised clots can be quite resistant to ward base bladder washout and irrigation. A GA cystoscopy and wash out allows the use of an Ellik evacuator to suck out resistant clots. If this is not successful, a resectoscope with a loop cutting element might be needed to break large organised clots up. After all clots have been removed, inspect the bladder for evidence of bleeding to control haemostasis.

Management of Haematuria Following Prostate Biopsy

Bleeding is a common consequence following needle biopsy of the prostate and can occur as haematospermia, rectal bleeding or haematuria, which is estimated to occurrence in up to two thirds of patients, and a fifth experiencing it for up to two weeks.. Most bleeding is self-limiting, but the need for hospitalisation can occur. Patients with Severe rectal bleeding must be resuscitated as described above, and can be treated with per rectal prostatic pressure, use of sponge enemas, a rectal pressure balloon catheter, or gauze soaked in 1:10,000 Adrenaline [10]. Severe haematuria can be treated as described above with the addition of catheter traction. If this fails, embolization should be considered (see below).

Management of Intractable Haematuria

Bladder Irrigants (Box 2)

Alum

Where initial measures fail to control haematuria, the use of bladder instillations may be helpful. Successful control of haematuria with the use of intravesical alum irrigation was first described by Ostroff and Chenault using a 1% alum solution in six patients without anaesthesia, and several case series with success of up to 100% have since been reported. [11]. Alum (aluminium ammonium sulphate or aluminium potassium sulphate) causes precipitation of proteins in the cell surface and interstitial spaces without cell necrosis, and without penetration of the full thickness of the bladder wall. The lack of anaesthetic requirement and apparent absence of serious complications make alum irrigation an attractive option for clinical practice. However, in reality, the authors have found Alum difficult to source in an emergency situation. The authors suggest that readers may like to find out where their closest supply of medical alum is for their institution to save time when it may be needed.

Silver Nitrate

Instillation of silver nitrate into the bladder causes coagulation and eschar at the sites of bleeding. A solution of 0.5% to 1.0% can be instilled for 10–20 minutes, and vesico-ureteric reflux (VUR) must first be excluded to prevent reflux of the solution causing coagulative obstruction of the ureters, which has been reported [12].

Formalin

Intravesical formalin irrigation is generally seen as a last resort following the failure of other methods on account of its potentially severe side effects. However, a number of cases have been reported of complete resolution of haematuria with a formalin solution in such patients [13]. Intravesical formalin treatment causes precipitation of cellular proteins of the bladder, and leads to occlusion and fixation of telangiectasia and small capillaries. However, severe side-effects have been described, including renal failure, reduction of bladder capacity, urinary incontinence, urgency and nocturia, and retroperitoneal fibrosis [14]. Formalin use can cause oedema, necrosis, and inflammation throughout all layers of the bladder. Furthermore, instillation is painful and requires general or spinal anaesthesia, and an irrigation catheter has to be left in the bladder after the procedure to control bleeding. Similarly to other instillations, cystoscopy and retrograde pyelogram should always be carried out before considering formalin treatment to remove blood clots and exclude VUR if VUR is present, ureteric occlusion catheters can be used to prevent the formalin solution from refluxing [15].

Box 2.

Protocols for various treatments [22]

Alum irrigation:
- Using a 1% alum solution; 50 g of alum is dissolved in 5 L sterile water and used to irrigate the bladder at 250±300 mL/h;
- Using the 1% solution or a stock solution of 400 g of potash of alum (McCarthy's) in 4 L hot sterile water; 300 mL of the stock solution is added to 3 L of 0.9% saline through a sterilizing filter and the bladder irrigated with up to 30 L of this solution in 24 h.

Intravesical formalin instillation:
- A low initial formalin concentration (1±2%) should be used, with progressively higher concentrations if necessary.
- Use cystography to exclude reflux; protect with a Fogarty catheter in the presence of reflux.
- Use spinal or general anaesthesia.
- Evacuate blood clots and coagulate major bleeding vessels.
- Protect all external areas on the skin and mucosa with Vaseline; pack the vagina to prevent leakage from catheter.
- Irrigate the bladder with a low concentration (1±2%) of formalin for 10 min under gravity at <15 cmH2O, or instil formalin under gravity at <15 cmH2O and leave the catheter open at a level just above the pubic ramus.
- Monitor the bladder pressure if possible and discontinue the procedure when the pressure is>50 cmH2O.
- Limit the contact time to 15 min.

Intravesical Prostaglandins:
Protocol 1
- Cystoscopy, clot evacuation and placement of a three-way 24 F Foley catheter.
- Instil 50 mL of 4±8 mg/L carboprost tromethamine in the bladder and maintain for 1 h.
- Drain the bladder, instil another 50 mL and maintain for 1 h.
- Unclamp the catheter and irrigate the bladder with normal saline.
- Repeat the carboprost tromethamine instillation four times a day.
- Each 24 h course consists of a total of 400 mL carboprost tromethamine for 8 h.
- If there is no improvement by courses 4±6, the dosage is increased to 10 mg/L.
Protocol 2
- Irrigate the bladder continuously with 8±10 mg/L carboprost tromethamine at 100 mL/h for 10 h.

Hydrodistension therapy:
- Use epidural anaesthesia;
- Use a Foley catheter and balloon or condom (as described);
- Fill the balloon or condom to 10±25 cmH2O above diastolic BP for 6 h.

Systemic Medication

Pentosan Polysulphate

Pentosan polysulphate is available on a named patient basis in the UK for the treatment of patients with haemorrhagic cystitis, which may result from radiotherapy for prostate cancer. Oral sodium pentosan polysulphate is reported to have no detectable anticoagulant activity, to be safe and not toxic, and therefore may be a useful adjunct in comorbid patients not fit for other treatments. It is thought that pentosan polysulphate helps to replenish the waterproof GAG layer of the bladder, which may be damaged by irradiation. A dose of 100 mg three times daily can be used, gradually reduced to a maintenance dose of 100 mg once daily, before stopping when bleeding ceases [16].

Epsilon-Aminocaproic Acid

Epsilon-Aminocaproic acid (EACA) is a synthetic lysin that competitively inhibits fibrinolysis. Fibrinolysis in the urinary tract is exacerbated by urokinases, which are present in urine, and can prevent clot formation at the site of bleeding vessels. EACA can be administered orally, parenterally, or intravesically via CBI and response rates of around 90% has been reported [17]. Reported side-effects of EACA are rare, but serious, including thrombotic complications, myopathy, rhabdomyolysis, and renal and hepatic failure [18]. When given orally, the drug is absorbed rapidly and most is secreted unchanged in the urine. For the intravenous regimen 4–5 g is given during the first hour of treatment, followed by a continuous infusion of 1 g/h , although total dose of EACA should not exceed 12 g per day because of the increased risk of thromboembolic events [19]. EACA (administered as 200 mg/l 0.9% in normal saline) can be instituted via continuous bladder irrigation. Before instillation therapy, all clots must be evacuated from the bladder as EACA may propagate the formation of hard clots that are not easily flushed from the bladder. Once the haematuria has resolved, irrigation should continue for an additional 24 h. This therapy is contraindicated in patients who have upper-tract bleeding, so it is important to localize the site of bleeding to the prostate and avoid acute renal failure due to obstruction.

5-α Reductase Inhibitors

The effectiveness of finasteride (an inhibitor of the formation of dihydrotestosterone responsible for BPH) in controlling haematuria associated with benign prostatic hyperplasia is well known. Given that many men with prostate cancer will also have a degree of benign enlargement of the prostate, such treatment may be effective for the treatment of haematuria in the context of prostate cancer. Finasteride has a slow onset of action (although one study suggested that vascular changes can be seen within two weeks) and therefore should be considered for use in chronic, not potentially life threatening haematuria. Dutasteride is a more potent inhibitor of 5-α reductase with a more rapid onset of action, which may give faster treatment of haematuria [20].

Degarelix

Degarelix is an antagonist of leuteonising hormone releasing hormone (LHRH), which is used for the treatment of advanced prostate cancer. In contrast to LHRH agonists, such as goserelin, or leuprorelin, which have traditionally been used for chemical castration in prostate cancer, Degarelix appears to have a more rapid onset of testosterone suppression (without the initial testosterone flare associated with LHRH agonists) achieving castrate levels within three days [21]. Degarelix is administered as a deep subcutaneous injection in the abdominal region with an initial dose of 240mg, followed by maintenance of 80mg every 28 days. Although the authors could find no literature on the use of Degarelix for the treatment of haematuria, they have found in their own practice to be a useful tool when treating patients with prostate cancer and intractable haematuria.

Hyperbaric Oxygen Therapy

The use of hyperbaric oxygen in the treatment of haematuria has long been used to reverse the cellular hypoxia caused by obliterative endarteritis of the small blood vessels of the bladder caused by radiotherapy.

Treatment of haematuria and avoidance of cystectomy have been prospectively demonstrated for patients with radiation cystitis and severe haematuria [22]. Hyperbaric oxygen therapy does not appear to promote cancer growth; and complications associated with barometric pressure changes or toxicity are rare, however, arduous regimens and the lack of facilities limit its use in clinical practice.

Hydrodistension (Box 2, Figure 3)

The use of intravesical hydrostatic pressure for the control of bladder haemorrhage was first described in 1972 by Helmstein using balloons inserted into the bladder via a catheter under epidural anaesthesia to render the bladder atonic [23].

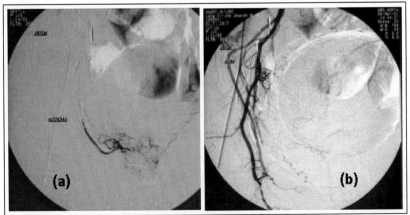

From: Rastinehad AR1, Caplin DM, Ost MC, VanderBrink BA, Lobko I, Badlani GH, Weiss GH, Kavoussi LR, Siegel DN. Selective arterial prostatic embolization (SAPE) for refractory haematuria of prostatic origin. Urology. 2008 Feb;71(2):181-4.

Figure 3. (a) Digital subtraction angiography of patient with refractory haematuria pre-embolization. (b) Digital subtraction angiography of patient with refractory haematuria post-embolization.

Initially intravesical pressures equivalent to systolic blood pressure for a period of up to 6 hours were used. Subsequent authors have described pressures at diastolic levels, on account of complications including bladder rupture, abdominal pain, nausea, temporary incontinence and pyrexia more commonly seen at higher pressure. Response rates of up to 100% have been reported, although limitations of the evidence base, plus the requirement for anaesthesia limit its usefulness in clinical practice.

Embolization

The first report of arterial embolization for the treatment of intractable haematuria was published in 1974 by Hald and Mygind, in which they reported unilateral hypogastric artery occlusion in a patient with bladder carcinoma. The authors described that bleeding stopped, but that side effects included tenderness and induration of the gluteal and posterior thigh region with urgency [24]. Technological advances in imaging, catheter equipment and embolization agents allow for selective embolization of fourth-order and fifth-order arterial branches. Selective arterial embolization for treatment of refractory prostatic bleeding in cases of prostate cancer has been described by Rastinehad et al., with successful treatment of haematuria in all eight patients within two days, lasting for follow-up of 20 months [25]. Similar results for the treatment of haematuria after pelvic irradiation for bladder and prostate cancer have also been reported. Complications resulting from the embolization of non-targeted areas can occur, tending to occur more frequently in cases of bleeding from pelvic trauma, and with less selective embolization. (Figure 4). Failure of percutaneous intervention may leave no choice other than open surgery with ligation of the internal iliac arteries.

Radiotherapy

Radiotherapy is a commonly used treatment for the palliation of chronic haematuria secondary to prostate cancer. A series by Gibbons et al. showed a reduction in haematuria in patients with locally advanced prostate cancer treated with radiotherapy [26]. More recent regimens of palliative radiotherapy for the treatment of prostate cancer typically involve a dose of 60 Gy in 2–3 Gy fractions, for 9 days a fortnight, which can induce an improvement in haematuria and overall symptoms.

Conclusion

Haematuria in the context of prostate cancer can be life threatening, it can be chronic, and it is often challenging to treat. Initial management involves resuscitation and catheterisation with washout and bladder irrigation. Failure of initial measures may require endoscopic management in theatre. If this fails then a combination of additional treatments may be necessary, which requires a multidisciplinary approach with haematologists, pharmacists, radiologists, and radiation oncologists. Careful consideration must also be given to any potential side effects or complications of unusual treatments, with which most urologists have infrequent experience.

References

[1]   Khadra MH, Pickard RS, Charlton M, Powell PH, Neal DE. A prospective analysis of 1930 patients with haematuria to evaluate current diagnostic practice. *J. Urol.* 2000 Feb; 163(2): 524-527.

[2]   Quantifying the risk of malignancy in patients with visible haematuria attending the Emergency Department, Marzouk S, Han Gan J, Harris A, Green JSA, BAUS 2012

[3]   Joint Consensus Statement on the Initial Assessment of Haematuria. http://www.baus.org.uk/Resources/BAUS/Documents/PDF%20Documents/BAUS%20i n%20general/haematuria_consensus_guidelines_July_2008.pdf

[4]   Hicks D, Li CY. Management of macroscopic haematuria in the emergency department. Emerg Med J 2007; 24: 385-390.

[5]   European Association of Urology Clinical Guidelines. http://www.uroweb.org/ guidelines/online-guidelines/

[6]   Braasch M, Antolak C, Hendlin K, Botnaru A, Herrera S, Lavers A, et al. Irrigation and drainage properties of three-way urethral catheters. *Urology.* 2006;67(1):40-4. Epub 2006/01/18.

[7]   Gravenstein D. Transurethral resection of the prostate (TURP) syndrome: a review of the pathophysiology and management. *Anesthesia and analgesia.* 1997;84(2):438-46. Epub 1997/02/01.

[8]   Warlick CA, Mouli SK, Allaf ME, Wagner AA, Kavoussi LR. Bladder irrigation using hydrogen peroxide for clot evacuation. *Urology.* 2006;68(6):1331-2. Epub 2006/12/16.

[9]   Bo J, Yangyang Y, Jiayuan L, Siwen D, Yong C, Junbo Y. Evaluation of bladder clots using a nonsurgical treatment. *Urology.* 2014;83(2):498-9. Epub 2013/12/10.

[10] Oxford Handbook of Urology. Eds. Reynard J, Brewster S, Biers S. Ch 7: Urological Neoplasia. P329. Oxford University Press. *Third Edition.* 2013. Oxford.

[11] Ostroff EB, Chenault OW Jr. Alum irrigation for the control of massive bladder hemorrhage. *J. Urol.* 1982; 128: 929±30.

[12] Ragavaiah NV and Soloway MS (1977) Anuria following silver nitrate irrigations for intractable bladder hemorrhage. *J. Urol.* 118: 681–682.

[13] Sarnack MJ et al. (1999) Intravesicular formaldehyde instillation and renal complications. *Clin. Nephrol* 51: 122–125

[14] Giannakopoulos X, Grammeniatis E, Chambilomatis P, Baltogiannis D. Massive haemorrhage of inoperable bladder carcinomas: treatment by intravesical formalin solution. *Int. Urol. Nephrol.* 1997; 29: 33–8.

[15] Choong SK, Walkden M, Kirby R. The management of intractable haematuria. *BJU Int.* 2000; 86: 951–9.

[16] Sandhu SS, Goldstraw M, Woodhouse CR. The management of haemorrhagic cystitis with sodium pentosan polysulphate. *BJU Int.* 2004 Oct;94(6):845-7.

[17] Stefanini M, English HA, Taylor AE. Safe and effective, prolonged administration of epsilon aminocaproic acid in bleeding from the urinary tract. *J. Urol.* 1990; 143: 559–61.

[18] Biswas CK, Milligan DA, Agte SD, Kenward DH, Tilley PJ. Acute renal failure and myopathy after treatment with aminocaproic acid. *Br. Med. J.* 1980; 28:115–16.

[19] Deysine M and Cliffton EE (1964) Mechanism of action of epsilon aminocaproic acid in the control of hemorrhage. *Ann. NY Acad. Sci.* 115: 291–297.

[20] Roehrborn CG, Boyle PJ, Nickel C, Hoefner K, Andriole G on behalf of the ARIA3001, ARIA3002 and ARIA3003 study investigators. Efficacy and safety of a dual inhibitor or 5-alpha-reductase types 1 and 2 (dutasteride) in men with benign prostatic hyperplasia. *Urology* 2002; 60:434-441.

[21] Klotz L, Boccon-Gibod L, Shore ND, et al. The efficacy and safety of degarelix: a 12-month, comparative, randomized, open-label, parallel-group phase III study in patients with prostate cancer. *BJU Int.* 2008;102(11):1531–1538.

[22] Bevers RFM, Bakker DJ, Kurth KH. Hyperbaric oxygen treatment for haemorrhagic radiation cystitis. *Lancet* 1995; 346: 803±5

[23] Helmstein K. Treatment of bladder carcinoma by a hydrostatic pressure technique. Report on 43 cases. *Br. J. Urol.* 1972; 44: 434–50.

[24] Hald T and Mygind T (1974) Control of life-threatening vesical hemorrhage by unilateral hypogastric artery muscle embolization. *J. Urol.* 112: 60–63.

[25] Rastinehad AR1, Caplin DM, Ost MC, VanderBrink BA, Lobko I, Badlani GH, Weiss GH, Kavoussi LR, Siegel DN. Selective arterial prostatic embolization (SAPE) for refractory haematuria of prostatic origin. *Urology.* 2008 Feb;71(2):181-4.

[26] Gibbons RP, Mason JT, Correa RJ Jr et al. Carcinoma of the prostate: local control with external beam radiotherapy. *J. Urol.* 1979; 121: 310–2.

In: Hematuria   ISBN: 978-1-63463-073-3
Editors: Nikhil Vasdev and G. Boustead   © 2015 Nova Science Publishers, Inc.

Chapter 17

Non-Visible Haematuria:
The Nephrologists' Role

Sandhya Seneviratne[*]

National Institute for Nephrology, Dialysis and Transplantation,
Jayantha Weerasekera Mawatha, Colombo, Sri Lanka

Introduction

Traditionally the first port of call for 'visible' or macroscopic haematuria, or blood in the urine evident to the naked eye, has been the urologist. 'Invisible' haematuria, or blood that is seen only when urine is examined under the microscope, is considered the domain of the nephrologist. A rather arbitrary criteria for referral when one considers that most macroscopic haematuria would have at one time been microscopic before the pathology became sufficiently gross to cause visible bleeding into the genitourinary tract. However, it must be acknowledged that the causes of haematuria that are amenable to surgical management do become evident as overt bleeding more readily than those causes originating from the kidney that are the purview of the nephrologist.

As has been oft said "a little blood goes a long way" and just 1ml of blood can cause a litre of urine to become red. Under normal circumstances a healthy individual excretes up to a million red blood cells in their urine a day. Therefore, 1 to 3 red corpuscles per high power field of spun urine is considered unremarkable in the absence of any other significant abnormality. Unlike macroscopic haematuria which the literature agrees almost always warrants further investigation, according to the current recommendations of most major organizations isolated microscopic haematuria to justify further investigation, either needs to be symptomatic or present in at least two of three clean catch mid-stream samples of urine taken over a period of ten days or longer [1,2]. For this reason, it is not generally recommended that asymptomatic individuals be screened for microscopic haematuria. As it is concentrated the first urine voided on waking is the best sample for evaluation of microscopic

---
[*] Corresponding author: Work Tel 0094-11-2422335/6, Email: sandhyaseneviratne@yahoo.com.

haematuria, however, for patient convenience, a random sample of urine is considered acceptable for general evaluation since red cells and casts tend to deteriorate with time specially if the specific gravity of urine is low or the pH of urine is high.

The further investigation of microscopic haematuria that resolves spontaneously is undertaken depending on the clinician's suspicion of the existence of significant pathology.

Causes of Haematuria

Bleeding can originate from anywhere along the genitourinary tract and therefore has a broad differential diagnosis. Below are listed some common causes of haematuria divided into two groups based on whether they are more likely to present as macroscopic or microscopic haematuria.

Table 1.

Macroscopic haematuria	Microscopic haematuria
Bladder cancer	Wilm's tumour, Renal cell carcinoma
Renal and bladder calculi	Hyperuricosuria, Hypercalciuria
Sloughed renal papillae	Renal artery thrombosis, Renal vein thrombosis
Renal cysts of any cause	Polycystic kidney disease, Medullary sponge kidney
Trauma	
Over anti-coagulation	
Arterio-venous malformations, Vesical varices	
Benign and malignant prostatic hyperplasia	
Left renal vein hypertension	
Cystitis, Prostatitis	Pyelonephritis
	Glomerulonephritis
Loin pain haematuria syndrome	Thin membrane disease
	IgA nephropathy
	Sickle cell trait, Sickle cell anaemia
	Alports's syndrome
	Schistosomiasis

Although the above list is not a comprehensive one, it does demonstrate that some of the diseases listed under those presenting as macroscopic haematuria could initially present as microscopic haematuria. The prevalence of microscopic haematuria varies based on the patient's age, gender and ethnicity and the diagnostic method used to identify microscopic haematuria in the studies conducted. The presence of risk factors, co-morbidities and presenting clinical symptoms and signs need also to be considered when deciding on how further work up should proceed.

Haemoglobinuria causing brown or red discolouration of the urine is sometimes considered interchangeably with haematuria, however this is not strictly correct and the causes of haemoglobinuria have not been included in the above list.

Table 2. Causes of brown/red discolouration of urine

Drugs	Food	Endogenous substances
Chloroquine	Fava beans	Red blood cells
Quinine	Beetroot	Haemoglobin
Metronidazole	Blackberries	Myoglobin
Rifampicin	Blueberries	Porphyrin
Nitrofurantoin	Artificial food colourings	Bilirubin
Sulfanamides	Paprika	Melanin
Desferrioxamine	Rhubarb	
Levodopa		
Methyldopa		
Phenytoin		
Prochloperazine		

Taking a History from a Patient with Red Urine: From a Nephrologists' Perspective

Red or brown discolouration of urine has many possible causes and it should not be assumed to be due to blood. It is useful to question the patient regarding the possible causes of red/brown discolouration of urine.

Depending on the population screened the presence of asymptomatic microscopic haematuria ranged from 0.19% to 21% [1]. Differences in the age and gender of patients screened account for these variations. Certain factors increase the risk of the patient having a 'nephrological' or renal cause of haematuria as opposed to a urological cause.

For instance younger female patients are more likely to have a nephrological cause of microscopic haematuria such as connective tissue diseases, thin membrane disease and medullary sponge kidney than older male patients with a history of smoking, exposure to certain chemicals or previous treatment with cyclophosphamide who are at risk for bladder cancer. Glomerular haematuria when visible tends be dark brown, cola coloured or smoky rather than the frank red colour often seen with urologic pathology and almost never form clots perhaps due to the presence of urokinase and tissue-type plasminogen activators in the glomeruli and in the renal tubules.

Fever, and dysuria suggest infection of the genito-urinary tract and loin pain in this setting suggests pyelonephritis.

A family history of renal disease especially cystic diseases and other inherited conditions such as thin membrane disease, if present, are often volunteered by patients themselves. A history of associated proteinuria and autoimmune conditions, presence of systemic symptoms such as joint involvement, night sweats and rashes, especially palpable maculo-papular vasculitic rashes, make a strong case for a significant renal involvement being present. A history of haemoptysis, nasal discharge, sinusitis and recurrent otitis media and hearing loss are features of reno-pulmonary syndromes which cause microscopic haematuria. Visual symptoms associated with hearing defects can be seen with Alport's syndrome. A preceding history of upper respiratory tract infections or gastroenteritis is associated with post-infectious glomerulonephritis and with IgA nephropathy. Abdominal pain associated with haematuria raises the possibility of Henoch-Schonlein Purpura especially in children. Asthma-like symptoms are features of certain vasculitides such as Churg-Strauss Syndrome that are associated with microscopic haematuria.

A history of hepatitis and ongoing endocarditis is also significant as these can cause immune-complex mediated glomerulonephritis. Anaemia from conditions such as sickle cell disease, living in areas endemic for schistosomiasis and living or having lived in areas endemic for certain renal conditions such as Balkan nephropathy and chronic kidney diseases of unknown origin such as that affecting the rural farming communities in Sri Lanka, are significant geographical features in the history suggesting a nephrological cause of haematuria. The ethnicity of the patient also makes certain conditions such as sickle cell disease related microscopic haematuria (Africans) and IgA nephropathy (Asians) more likely.

Anticoagulation per se is not a cause for haematuria unless there is bleeding from multiple sites due to over anti-coagulation. A history of coagulopathy need to be elicited. It is generally recommended that isolated haematuria in those on anti-coagulation be evaluated in the same manner as those not on anti-coagulation [3]. Use of drugs such as analgesics is associated with interstitial nephritis and microscopic haematuria.

Microscopic haematuria may also be transient and may sometimes be seen in post menopausal women[4]. The cause for transient microscopic haematuria is often not clear. Contamination of urine with menstrual blood, following vigorous exercise, sexual intercourse and mild trauma are benign causes of transient microscopic haematuria that can be diagnosed by taking a detailed history. The microhaematuria should resolve forty-eight hours after cessation of the precipitating activity [2].

Although the differential diagnosis is broad, from the history alone it is possible to gauge to a fair extent the possible aetiology of the condition affecting the kidney and causing microscopic haematuria. Approximately fifty percent of patients with idiopathic haematuria have a glomerular disease [5] and overall the commonest nephrological cause for isolated haematuria is probably IgA nephropathy [6] with thin membrane disease being nearly as frequent [7].

Physical Examination

A careful physical examination of the patient will alert the astute physician and save much time and expense by guiding the line of investigation to pursue.

The examination could reveal oedema, scratch marks, anaemia and dry 'frosty' skin which are compatible with established renal impairment of any cause. Jaundice would suggest hepatitis causing an associated immune-complex mediated glomerulonephritis such as mesangiocapillary or membranoproliferative glomerulonephritis. In tropical countries and in farming communities in developed countries the presence of jaundice, conjunctival suffusion and acute renal failure with petichae would suggest leptospirosis infection with the passage of dark urine being due to bilirubin as well as haematuria which could be microscopic rather than frank. The urine sediment in hepato-renal syndrome it must be remembered is unremarkable. The presence of hypertension with or without signs of renal impairment, scleritis and uveitis, strongly suggest a glomerular cause of haematuria due to autoimmune diseases. Similarly, the presence of typical rashes of systemic lupus erythematosus, vasculitic rashes and subcutaneous nodules also suggest collagen vascular diseases. Bruits over the kidneys suggest a vascular cause and atrial fibrillation raises the possibility of renal emboli causing micro infarcts and microscopic haematuria.

Investigating Microscopic Haematuria

The nephrologist is interested in determining whether the microscopic haematuria originates from the kidneys or not. Therefore the aetiologies considered in the history and examination is rationally categorized into those affecting the various elements of the kidney and investigation and analysis of findings follow. A more useful classification of haematuria from the nephrologists' diagnostic point of view is probably that given below which identifies the sites of bleeding due to the various diseases rather than on whether they are more likely to present as microscopic haematuria or macroscopic haematuria at the initial presentation.

Sources of Haematuria

Glomerular	Tubulo Interstitial	Vascular
IgA nephropathy	Renal cystic diseases	Coagulopathies
Thin membrane disease	Interstitial nephritis	Over anti-coagulation
Alport's syndrome	Analgesic nephropathy	Arterial thrombosis and embolisation
Primary glomerulonephritis	Tuberculosis	Renal vein thrombosis
Secondary glomerulonephritis	Pyelonephritis	Arterio-venous malformations
Fabry's disease	Hereditary nephritis	Nutcracker syndrome
		Loin-pain haematuria syndrome
Multiple sites	**Urothelium**	
Hypercalciuria	Vigorous exercise	
Hyperuricosuria	Trauma	
Sickle cell disease	Malignancy	
	Renal calculi	
	Prostatitis/Urethritis/Cystitis	
	Papillary necrosis	
	Schistosomiasis	

The simplest test used to screen for microscopic haematuria is the urine dipstick test, which is a test for reducing substances. This will give a positive result not only when whole red blood cells are present but also in the presence of free haemoglobin and myoglobin (haemoglobinuria or myoglobinuria), ascorbic acid (>5 mg per deciliter) or antiseptic povidone–iodine as well as certain other reducing substances. When dipstick testing of urine gives a positive result microscopy is carried out to differentiate the presence of whole red cells from haem and globin pigments. Unlike the presence of pigments which would suggest haemolysis or rhabdomyolysis, the presence of whole red cells in significant numbers must originate from the genitourinary tract. The urine should be tested for evidence of urinary tract infection and if nitrites, bacteruria or pyuria is present, should be treated appropriately for urinary tract infection. Urinalysis should be repeated six weeks later and if haematuria has resolved no further evaluation is undertaken [3].

The presence of dysmorphic red cells in urine has traditionally been considered a marker of glomerular bleeding. The percentage of dysmorphic red cells (cells of varying size with blebs, budding and protrusions) needed to classify bleeding as being of glomerular origin has not been well defined. More than eighty percent of red cells being dysmorphic are highly suggestive of being of glomerular origin provided a fresh sample of urine is examined. More than eighty percent of cells being normal suggest lower tract bleeding. Percentages falling in between these two could indicate bleeding from either source [8, 9]. For practical purposes the presence of acanthocytes (red cells with vesicle-shaped protrusions "Mickey Mouse ears") are much more specific and if more than five percent of red cells are thus affected is very suggestive of glomerular bleeding [10].

A comprehensive analysis of the urine sediment should be undertaken and the presence and type of casts and the presence and degree of proteinuria noted. Blood originating from the glomeruli are subject to changes in osmolality, pH, ionic strengths and other forces as they pass along the tubules. The red cells also get compressed together with Tamm-Horsfall urinary proteins in the distal tubules and form red cell casts which if seen in the urine are an excellent indicator of glomerular bleeding. White cell casts are often indicative of interstitial nephritis but can be seen in glomerulonephritis as well.

The most important indicator of glomerular origin of bleeding and glomerular damage is the presence of proteinuria. When the screening urine dipstick test becomes positive for urinary protein a quantitative analysis is carried out. However with very high urine outputs significant proteinuria may not be detected on dipstick testing due to dilution. Ideally a timed 24-hour urine collection should be carried out to quantify the proteinuria at least initially. A spot sample of urine for urine albumin:creatinine ratio is an acceptable alternative especially for follow up of treatment. More than 300mg a day of proteinuria points to glomerular protein leak, 500mg a day of proteinuria is significant [11] and more than 1g a day in the absence of massive bleeding would be unlikely to be from any other site than the glomeruli and further investigations would be focused on the glomerular causes of haematuria [12]. These tests would include serological tests such as immunological screening for anti-nuclear antibodies, antibodies to double-stranded DNA, anti Smith and anti-Rho antibodies for lupus nephritis and collagen vascular diseases. The presence of anti-neutrophil cytoplasmic antibodies (MPO and PR3 antibodies) helps establish a diagnosis of vasculitis and anti-glomerular basement membrane antibodies a diagnosis of Goodpasture's syndrome. Complement C3 and C4 levels can be normal or low depending on the cause of glomerulonephritis and C3 nephritic factor is seen in mesangiocapillary glomerulonephritis type II. Serum IgA levels are sometimes raised in IgA nephropathy. Hepatitis and HIV serology, echocardiography, anti-streptolysin O titres for post-infectious glomerulonephritis and blood cultures are also done to look for secondary glomerulonephritides. The importance of the detailed history and clinical findings on examination becomes evident when one considers the above list of potential investigations and diagnostic pathways. The differential diagnosis must guide which investigations would be indicated as clearly it would be irrational and expensive to embark on a series of undirected tests.

The presence of other formed elements in the urine can give useful indicators of rarer causes of microscopic haematuria. For instance calcium oxalate crystals and urate crystal suggest hypercalciuria and uricosuria associated microscopic haematuria respectively and nephrolithiasis. Timed 24-hour urinary calcium and urate excretions can confirm these. The presence of eosinophils in the urine suggests allergic interstitial nephritis and analgesic nephropathy as a cause of microscopic haematuria.

Next to proteinuria the assessment of renal function is probably the most productive investigation in terms of defining further investigations, diagnosis and treatment of microscopic haematuria from a nephrologists' perspective. Significantly impaired renal function is fairly easily detected with a serum creatinine level and together with haematuria mandates early and vigorous work-up of the patient. When haematuria is associated with significant proteinuria and renal impairment, especially if renal impairment is acute, a rapidly progressive glomerulonephritis must be speedily investigated for and treated. This includes the previously discussed immunological markers as well as other biochemical tests needed for the day to day management of the patient. A renal biopsy also needs to be speedily carried out in this setting.

Ultrasonographic imaging of the 'renal' patient has become one of the very early tests recommended for most renal conditions. It is necessary to verify the normal position and sizes of the kidneys, the presence of both kidneys and the absence of significant anatomical variations prior to undertaking a renal biopsy. Also, conditions such as polycystic kidneys giving rise to haematuria are easily diagnosed and large tumours can be seen . Similarly renal calculi and nephrocalcinosis can often be seen on a simple ultrasound. Medullary sponge kidneys are better visualized on an intravenousurogram as are the rarer arteriovenous malformations and smaller renal tumours that may give rise to microhaematuria. Doppler of the renal vasculature can provide information as to the state of the renal blood flow, however a computed tomographic renal angiogram is now considered the gold-standard for visualizing the renal vasculature. It will also show any tumours, abscesses and other anatomical lesions.

Management Strategies in Microscopic Haematuria

The essential questions to which the nephrologist seeks answers are whether the haematuria is truly originating from the kidneys or elsewhere in the urogenital tract and whether a neoplastic lesion is the cause.

If no diagnosis can be made from the history, physical signs, imaging, cystoscopy and urinalysis as to the cause of persistent isolated microscopic haematuria the most likely cause is probably a mild glomerulopathy or a predisposition to stone disease with hypercalciuria or hyperuricosuria [13]. Treatment of hypercalciuria with a thiazide and of uricosuria with allopurinol is generally recommended and the haematuria has often been shown to disappear. However in some series upto 9.4% of patients with microscopic haematuria were found to have neoplasms [14].

Since no cause of isolated microscopic haematuria in the absence of any other symptoms, signs or positive basic investigations needs urgent diagnosis or treatment it is reasonable to repeat the urinalysis to see whether the microhaematuria disappears. Transient isolated microscopic haematuria is a common problem in adults [15] and often no aetiology can be identified. An important exception is older adults, those with risk factors for malignancy and those with intermittent microscopic haematuria on dipstick. These patients, provided no glomerular bleeding is identified, need further imaging of the upper tract and workup including urine cytology and cystoscopy.

Isolated glomerular microhaematuria in the absence of renal impairment and proteinuria does not require renal biopsy as the biopsy result is unlikely to change the clinical management[16]. These patients are usually followed up regularly in a renal clinic monitoring for deterioration of renal function, or the emergence of any new significant symptoms, signs or investigation results such as gross haematuria, hypertension, proteinuria or abnormal urine cytology. The most likely diagnosis in this group of patients is likely to be IgA nephropathy or thin membrane disease.

Patients with microscopic haematuria with active urinary sediment, proteinuria, renal impairment and rising blood pressure require a renal biopsy as part of their evaluation in addition to the serological investigations discussed previously. Those patients with isolated microscopic haematuria being monitored also need a renal biopsy should they develop any such significant features.

The management of rapidly progressive glomerulonephritis can be considered a nephrological emergency. The treatment involves plasma exchange, high dose methyl prednisolone and cytotoxic drugs such as cyclophosphamide. The patient may need dialysis for renal failure, counseling to administer cytotoxic drugs, storage of sperm and ova and ventilatory support. They are best managed in a tertiary renal referral centre with access to a multidisciplinary team.

Treatment of specific glomerulonephritides depends on the type of glomerulonephritis and on whether it is primary or secondary. The essential strategy requires some form of immunosuppressive treatment unless it is secondary to an ongoing infection such as endocarditis. The optimum type and duration of treatment varies and are usually based on current multi-centre trial data.

Certain causes of microscopic haematuria such as cystic kidney disease are progressive and unfortunately could end in renal failure. The strategy here is to counsel early and arrange a renal transplant once the patient reaches end-stage renal failure.

Avoiding long-term use of non-steroidal anti-inflammatory drugs, is good policy not only for those with allergic nephritis but for all patients. Steroids have been shown to be useful in allergic nephritis [17]. Renal tuberculosis requires a prolonged course of treatment including steroids and anti-tuberculous antibiotics. The recommended treatment regimens are different in various parts of the world depending on drug sensitivity patterns local to the region. Specific treatment of other conditions such as arterio-venous malformations evolves from time to time. At present radiological embolisation is the preferred mode of minimally invasive therapy. Correction of coagulopathies and anti-coagulation of thromboembolism is according to the current standard practices.

References

[1]   Gary, D., Grossfeld, J., Stuart Wolf, Jr., Mark, S., Litwin, Hedvig Hricak, Cathryn, L., Shuler, David, C. & Agerter, Peter, R. (2001). Carroll, Asymptomatic Microscopic Hematuria in Adults: Summary of the AUA Best Practice Policy Recommendations, *Am Fam Physician.* Mar 15, *63*(6), 1145-1155.

[2]   McDonald, M., Swagerty, D. & Wetzel, L. (2006). Assessment of Microscopic Hematuria in Adults. *American Family Physician*, *73*(10), 1748-1754.

[3]   Avidor, Y., et al. (2000). Clinical significance of gross hematuria and its evaluation in patients receiving anticoagulant and aspirin treatment. *Urology.* January, *55*, 22–4.

[4]   Mohr, D. N., Offord, K. P., Owen, R. A. & Melton, L. J. III. (1986). Asymptomatic microhematuria and urologic disease: a population-based study. *JAMA*, *256*, 224-229

[5]   Topham, P. S., Harper, S. J., Furness, P. N., et al. (1994). Glomerular disease as a cause of isolated microscopic microscopic haematuria. *Q J Med*, *87*, 329.

[6]   Tanaka, H., Kim, S. T., Takasugi, M. & Kuroiwa (1996). Isolated hematuria in adults: IgA nephropathy is a predominant cause of hematuria compared with thin glomerular basement membrane nephropathy. *Am J Nephr*, *15*(5), 412-6.

[7]   Nieuwhof, C., Doorenbos, C., Grave, W., et al. (1996). A prospective study of the natural history of idiopathic non-proteinuric hematuria. *Kidney Int.*, *49*, 222.

[8]   Pollock, C., Liu, P. L., Gyory, A. Z., Grigg, R., Gallery, E. D., Caterson, R., et al. (1989). Dysmorphism of urinary red blood cells—value in diagnosis. *Kidney Int.*, *36*, 1045–9.

[9]   De Santo, N. G., Nuzzi, F., Capodicasa, G., Lama, G., Caputo, G., Rosati, P., et al. (1987). Phase contrast microscopy of the urine sediment for the diagnosis of glomerular and nonglomerular bleeding—data in children and adults with normal creatinine clearance. *Nephron.*, *45*, 35–9.

[10]   Köhler, H., Wandel, E. & Brunck, B. (1991). Acanthocyturia--a characteristic marker for glomerular bleeding., *Kidney Int.*, Jul, *40*(1), 115-20.

[11]   Robert, A. (2003). Cohen, Robert S. Brown, Microscopic Hematuria, *N Engl J Med.*, *348*, 2330-2338 June 5.

[12]   Tapp, D. C. & Copley, J. B. (1988) Effect of red blood cell lysis on protein quantitation in hematuric states. *Am J Nephrol.*, *8*, 190–3.

[13]   Andres, A., Praga, M., Bello, I., et al. (1989) Hematuria due to hypercalciuria and hyperuricosuria in adult patients. *Kidney Int*, *36*, 96-99.

[14]   Khadra, M. H., Pickard, R. S., Charlton, M., Powell, P. H. & Neal, D. E. (2000). A prospective analysis of 1,930 patients with hematuria to evaluate current diagnostic practice. *J Urol.*, *163*, 524–7.

[15]   Froom, P., Ribak, J. & Benbassat, J. (1984). Significance of microhaematuria in young adults. *Br Med J.*, *288*, 20.

[16]   McGregor, D. O., Lynn, K. L., Bailey, R. R., Robson, R. A. & Gardner, J. (1998). Clinical audit of the use of renal biopsy in the management of isolated microscopic hematuria. *Clin Nephrol*, *49*, 345-8.

[17]   Jeffrey Ricketson, Gil Kimel, James Spence, Rene Weir (2009). Acute allergic interstitial nephritis after use of pantoprazole *CMAJ*, March 3, vol. *180*, no. 5.

In: Hematuria
Editors: Nikhil Vasdev and G. Boustead

ISBN: 978-1-63463-073-3
© 2015 Nova Science Publishers, Inc.

Chapter 18

Hematuria and Trauma

Qing Hui Wu* and Kesavan Esuvaranathan

Department of Urology, National University Hospital, Singapore

Injuries to the genitourinary tract can involve the kidneys, ureters, bladder, urethra, and external genitalia. About 10% of all injuries in the emergency room are genitourinary injuries. The most commonly injured organ is the kidney; the second is the urethra and the third is the bladder.

1. Renal Trauma

1.1. Etiology

Because of its relatively protected position, a considerable degree of force is usually required to cause a kidney injury. Therefore there may be associated injuries to, for example, the spleen, liver, mesentery of the bowel, or other organs. In children, there is proportionately less perirenal fat to cushion the kidneys against injury, and thus renal injuries occur with lesser degrees of trauma. Kidneys with existing pathologic conditions such as hydronephrosis or malignant tumors are also more readily ruptured from mild trauma.

There are two broad categories of renal injury— blunt and penetrating injury. Blunt injuries occur either as a result of a direct blow to the kidney or a rapid acceleration or deceleration. They account for 80~85% of all renal injuries. The commonest causes of blunt renal injuries in urban societies are motor vehicle accidents, falls, assaults and contact sports.

Hematuria is a hallmark sign of renal injury, but is neither sensitive nor specific enough for differentiating minor and major injuries. The degree of hematuria and the grade of renal injury, however, did not correlate. Major renal injury may occur without hematuria. In a deceleration injury, for example, both the intima of the renal artery and the ureteropelvic

---
* Corresponding author: Email: qing_hui_wu@nuhs.edu.sg.

junction are susceptible to tearing, resulting in arterial thrombosis or disruption of the ureteropelvic junction. However, this can occur without any hematuria. One study in blunt renal trauma showed Grade 2 to 4 renal injuries had microscopic hematuria and no shock in 8.3% and no hematuria in 20.8% of the patients. In a study by Eastham in patients with stab wounds, 9% of patients with stab wounds and resultant proven renal injury did not manifest hematuria. Hematuria out of proportion to the history of trauma suggests pre-existing renal pathology. A urine dipstick is a rapid and reliable test to screen for microscopic hematuria; however, false-negative findings do occur in approximately 2.5-10% of cases.

1.2. Investigation

Adult patients with a history of blunt trauma and microscopic hematuria need not have their kidneys imaged as long as there is no history of acceleration/deceleration and no shock, since the chances of a significant injury being found are <0.2%. The clinician should continue to maintain a low threshold for renal imaging in the pediatric population.

Renal imaging should be performed when:

- Macroscopic hematuria
- Penetrating chest, flank, and abdominal wounds
- Microscopic hematuria in a hypotensive patient
- A history of a rapid acceleration or deceleration
- Any child with microscopic hematuria who has sustained trauma

Although an intravenous pyelogram (IVP) is still considered useful in the evaluation of the suspected upper tracts injuries, it has been replaced by the contrast-enhanced CT scan as the imaging study of choice in most of the centers. It provides accurate information about depth and extent of lacerations, a functioning contralateral kidney, the presence of associated hematoma and contrast extravasation any devitalized renal parenchyma as well as other concomitant injuries in other organs.

Ultrasound can establish the presence of a retroperitoneal hematoma and with power Doppler can identify the presence of blood flow in the renal vessels. However, it cannot accurately identify parenchymal tears, collecting system injuries, or extravasation of urine until a later. Therefore, it is seldom used as the primary imaging modality. Screening with ultrasound may eliminate unnecessary CT scans.

Where a patient is transferred immediately to the operating theatre without having had a CT scan due to unstable conditions, evaluation of the kidneys may be accomplished by injecting intravenous contrast when the patient is under anesthesia and taking an abdominal x-ray 5–10 minutes after contrast administration (2 mL/kg of contrast) on the operating room table (one-shot IVP). It is proven useful in deciding the need for renal exploration when a retroperitoneal hematoma is found. On-table IVP can also be very helpful in determining the presence of a normally functioning contralateral kidney where the injury to the ipsilateral kidney is likely to necessitate a nephrectomy.

Grade	Description
I	Contusion (normal CT) or subcapsular haematoma with no parenchymal laceration
II	<1 cm deep parenchymal laceration of cortex, no extravasation of urine (i.e., collecting system intact)
III	>1 cm deep parenchymal laceration of cortex, no extravasation of urine (i.e., collecting system intact)
IV	Parenchymal laceration involving cortex, medulla, and collecting system, *or* renal artery or renal vein injury with contained haemorrhage
V	Completely shattered kidney *or* avulsion of renal hilum

Figure 1. Organ injury scaling classification of kidney injuries.

Using CT, renal injuries can be graded according to the American Association for the Surgery of Trauma (AAST) Organ Injury Severity Scale (Figure 1). The scale correlates with patient outcomes and permits appropriate and selective management to be undertaken.

1.3. Management

In recent years, advances in staging techniques resulting from increased use of CT scan as well as increased awareness of the kidney's capacity for healing have permitted the majority of these injuries to be successfully managed nonoperatively.

Over 95% of blunt injuries can be managed conservatively. In a recent series of grade IV lacerations at San Francisco General Hospital, 22% were successfully managed nonoperatively. Penetrating injuries more commonly require laparotomy because of associated injuries or hemodynamic instability. In our experience, however, 55% of stab wounds and 24% of gunshot wounds were successfully managed expectantly using careful selection and complete clinical and radiographic staging. If expectant management is selected for a major renal laceration, close monitoring with serial hematocrit measurements and liberal use of repeat imaging are indicated. The expectant approach thus does not imply nonsurgical management, and the urologist must be prepared to intervene surgically when necessary.

High-grade (IV and V) injuries can also be managed nonoperatively, as long as the patient is cardiovascularly stable. Urinary extravasation is not in itself necessarily an indication for exploration. Almost 90% of these injuries can heal spontaneously. Serial CT scans are mandatory in the management of these patients. The first scan should be obtained at approx 36–48 h post-injury to rule out the development of significant new complications. Intervention is indicated for sepsis, ongoing leakage, or significant urinoma formation. In these cases, placement of an indwelling ureteral (double J) stent may speed resolution of extravasation. Lacerations of the renal pelvis or UPJ avulsion usually do not resolve spontaneously and should be surgically repaired. In a study by Long, in the patients with urine extravasation from blunt trauma, ureteric stent placement and open surgery was required in 37% and 15% of patients, respectively. They also showed that a devascularised parenchyma volume of > 25% predicts a higher rate of surgery and poorer renal function.

In general terms, renal exploration is indicated for: persistent bleeding (persistent tachycardia and/or hypotension failing to respond to appropriate fluid and blood replacement), expanding perirenal hematoma, pulsatile perirenal hematoma. For the approach to renal exploration, the injury should be explored through a midline transperitoneal incision. most surgeons will elect to approach the renal pedicle first to allow control of the renal artery and vein. After lifting the small bowel upward to allow access to the retroperitoneum, Incision was made at the peritoneum over the aorta, above the inferior mesenteric artery or medial to the inferior mesenteric vein if a large retroperitoneal hematoma obviates easy palpation of the aorta. Once on the aorta, the inferior vena cava may be exposed, then the renal veins and the renal arteries. After passing slings around all of these vessels to allow control of bleeding, the kidney can now be exposed by mobilizing the colon.

Despite the ongoing advances in trauma care, successful renal salvage after major renovascular injury only occurs in 25 to 35% of cases. A recent multicenter review of outcomes following Grade V injury found that attempted arterial repair correlated with a poor result (renovascular hypertension, renal dysfunction). Therefore, we should reserve renal arterial repair for solitary kidneys, bilaterally injured kidneys, and within 6 h of injury. In all other cases, nephrectomy appears to be the treatment of choice. Arteriography with selective renal embolization for hemorrhage control is a reasonable alternative to laparotomy provided no other indication for immediate surgery exists.

1.4. Prognosis

Delayed retroperitoneal bleeding can occur within several weeks of the injury, and is managed with selective angiographic embolization. Perinephric abscess formation can be managed with percutaneous drainage, which has a lower rate of renal loss than open reoperation and drainage. Hypertension after renal trauma is estimated to occur in less than 5% of patients, and is caused acutely by external compression from a perirenal hematoma or chronically as a result of compressive scar formation. Treatment includes pharmacological management, excision of ischemic parenchyma, vascular reconstruction, or nephrectomy.

Urinary extravasation usually resolves over time unless obstruction or infection is present. Persistent extravasation usually responds well to stent placement or nephrostomy drainage.

2. Urethral Trauma

Urethral injuries mainly happen in the males. The male urethra is divided into the anterior and posterior sections by the urogenital diaphragm. The posterior urethra consists of the prostatic and the membranous urethra. The anterior urethra consists of the bulbar and penile urethra.

Type	Description	Appearance
I	Contusion	Blood at the urethral meatus; normal urethrogram
II	Stretch injury	Elongation of the urethra without extravasation on urethrography
III	Partial disruption	Extravasation of contrast at injury site with contrast visualized in the bladder
IV	Complete disruption	Extravasation of contrast at injury site without visualization in the bladder; <2 cm of urethral separation
V	Complete disruption	Complete transection with >2 cm urethral separation, or extension into the prostate or vagina

Figure 2. Organ injury scaling classification of urethral injuries.

AAST proposed the classification given in Figure 2.

2.1. Etiology

Anterior urethral injuries result from blunt trauma more frequently than from penetrating trauma. Most anterior urethral injuries are caused by vehicle accidents, falls, or blows; in contrast to posterior urethral trauma, they are rarely associated with pelvic fractures. The incidence of anterior urethral injuries is low, comprising only 10% of lower urinary tract injuries. Of these, bulbar urethral injuries comprise 85%. Blunt trauma typically affects the bulbar urethra as a result of a straddle injury from a fall, crush, or motor vehicle accident against the perineum. Pendulous urethral injury occurs in 15 to 37% of penile fractures, which usually occurs during intercourse.

Injuries to the posterior urethra occur with pelvic fractures, which are commonly caused by road traffic accidents, crush injuries, or falls from height. Overall, the male posterior urethra is concomitantly injured in approximately 3.5%–19% and the female urethra in 0%–6% of all pelvic fractures.

The following clinical indicators of acute urethral trauma warrant a complete urethral evaluation:

1. Blood at the Meatus

Blood at the meatus is present in 37%–93% of patients with posterior urethral injury and at least 75% of patients with anterior urethral trauma. Its presence should preclude any attempts at urethral instrumentation, until the entire urethra is adequately imaged. If a urethral injury is suspected, urethrography prior to attempted catheterization is the most prudent approach.

2. Blood at the Vaginal Introitus

Blood at the vaginal introitus is present in more than 80% of female patients with pelvic fractures and co-existing urethral injuries.

3. Hematuria

Although nonspecific, hematuria on a first voided specimen may indicate urethral injury. The amount of urethral bleeding correlates poorly with the severity of injury, as a mucosal contusion or small partial tear may be accompanied by copious bleeding, while total transection of the urethra may result in little bleeding.

4. Pain on Urination or Inability to Void

The inability to void suggests urethral disruption.

5. Hematoma or Swelling

With anterior urethral trauma, the pattern of the hematoma can be useful in identifying the anatomical boundaries violated by the injury. Extravasation of blood or urine in a sleeve distribution along the penile shaft indicates that the injury is confined by Buck's fascia. Disruption of Buck's fascia results in a pattern of extravasation limited only by Colles fascia, extending therefore up to the coracoclavicular fascia superiorly and the fascia lata inferiorly. This results in a characteristic butterfly pattern of bruising in the perineum.

6. High Riding Prostate

This is a relatively unreliable finding in the acute phase, since the pelvic hematoma associated with pelvic fractures often precludes the adequate palpation of the prostate.

2.2. Investigations

In trauma setting, often the CT scan finding of an inferomedial pubic bone fracture or symphysis diastasis predicts urethral injury with a sensitivity of 92% and specificity of 64%.

Retrograde urethrography is considered the gold standard for evaluating urethral injury. If posterior urethral injury is suspected, a suprapubic catheter is inserted; a simultaneous cystogram and ascending urethrogram can be carried out at a later date to assess the site, severity, and length of the urethral injury. When the proximal urethra is not visualized in a simultaneous cystogram and urethrogram, flexible cystoscopy through the suprapubic tract can be used to define the anatomy of the posterior urethra. Magnetic resonance imaging can provide additional information in selected complex or reoperative cases.

2.3. Management

Management of contusions is straightforward, consisting of urethral catheterization alone. The catheter is removed 10 to 14 d after injury and is followed by voiding cystourethrography at the time of removal. The management of more severe urethral injuries remains controversial due to the variety of injury patterns, associated injuries, treatment options available and lack randomized prospective studies.

2.3.1. Anterior urethral trauma

The best management is simply suprapubic diversion. The cystostomy tube is maintained for approximately 4 weeks to allow urethral healing. Voiding cystourethrography is then performed and if normal voiding can be reestablished. Satisfactory urethral luminal recanalization occurs in approximately 50% of partial anterior urethral disruptions. Short and flimsy strictures can be managed with optical urethrotomy or urethral dilation. Denser strictures require formal urethral reconstruction.

Repair of a traumatic stricture should be delayed at least 2 months after the initial injury. Bulbar urethral strictures shorter than 2.5 cm are usually amenable to resection and primary end-to-end anastomosis. Strictures of the pendulous urethra and those in the bulbar urethra that are longer than 2.5 cm will likely require substitution urethroplasty with a flap or graft.

2.3.2. Posterior urethral trauma

The triad of urinary retention, blood at the meatus, and high-riding prostate is the classic presentation of patients with injuries to the posterior urethra, present in 91%, 87%, and 64% of these patients, respectively.

Initial management depends on the patient's hemodynamic stability and the status of associated orthopedic and nonorthopedic injuries. Two options now exist for the management of posterior urethral injury: primary realignment or suprapubic cystostomy with delayed repair. Endoscopic realignment can be performed as soon as the patient is stabilized, although results still controversial. In one large study showed that patient who underwent endoscopic realignment developed less clinically significant strictures that required perineal urethroplasty and also experienced a slightly lower incidence of impotence and incontinence than the delayed reconstruction group.

Posterior urethroplasty is delayed until it can be performed under ideal conditions. A perineal approach is adequate in most cases; transpubic procedures are reserved for complex or reoperative cases in which a tension-free bulboprostatic anastomosis is not otherwise possible. Complete resection of the fibrotic segment with end-to-end anastomosis is the most successful method for posterior urethral reconstruction. Distal urethral mobilization is routinely accomplished to the level of the suspensory ligament of the penis. If necessary, corporal body separation, inferior pubectomy, or supracrural urethral rerouting may be utilized in sequential fashion to bridge the defect.

Erectile dysfunction occurs in 20%–60% of patients after traumatic posterior urethral rupture. Available data suggest that the severity of the initial injury is the most important determining factor associated with impotence.

3. Bladder Trauma

In the adult, the bladder lies in the true pelvis and, when not grossly distended, is well protected from injury. The 2002 Consensus Statement on Bladder Injuries categorizes these injuries based on appearance of the cystogram: contusion (usually a mucosal or muscularis injury without extravasation), intraperitoneal rupture, extraperitoneal rupture, and combined intraand extraperitoneal rupture.

Intraperitoneal bladder rupture occurs in a fully distended bladder because the sudden increase in intravesical pressure from blunt lower abdominal trauma. In contrast, extraperitoneal bladder injuries are nearly always associated with pelvic fracture.

Gross hematuria is the hallmark sign of injury to the bladder, present in greater than 95% of bladder ruptures from both blunt and penetrating injury; clinical findings can include suprapubic pain, dysuria, ileus, or an acute abdomen. Suspected bladder injury warrants conventional cystography or CT cystography. When performed properly, either imaging technique is highly sensitive and specific in identifying bladder injury.

As long as the patient has uninfected urine and appropriate catheter care, all patients with an extraperitoneal bladder injury can be managed with large-bore suprapubic or Foley catheter placed and should be maintained on prophylactic. Spontaneous healing occurs in 74 to 87% of patients after 2 weeks of bladder rest. Another 11 to 13% will heal with prolonged drainage for 2 to 13 weeks. Formal repair is indicated if there are any complicating features, such as the presence of vaginal or rectal injuries, lacerations that extend into the bladder neck, open pelvic fracture, or bony fragments projecting into the bladder.

All intraperitoneal bladder ruptures should be explored through either a lower midline incision or a formal laparotomy incision if other intraabdominal injury is suspected. The dome of the bladder should be opened via a midline cystotomy, and the bladder mucosa should be inspected. Each ureteral orifice should be inspected for signs of injury.

After bladder injury repair, long-term voiding dysfunction is usually not significant. The most common complications after repair include urinary tract infections and bladder spasms. However, more severe complications can occur, including incontinence, abscess formation, or fistula.

4. Ureter Trauma

Ureteral injuries constitute 1- 3% of all genitourinary injuries from external trauma. The ureter's mobility and anatomic characteristics protect it from trauma; its narrow diameter and retroperitoneal location between major muscle groups and the spine make it an unlikely target. They typically result from gunshot wounds, with blunt trauma and stab wounds responsible for less than 20% of ureteral injuries. Hematuria (gross or microscopic) is unreliable, as it is absent in about 26% of cases. Ureteral injuries from blunt trauma are rare. They usually occur in children or young adults during rapid deceleration, which causes disruption at the ureteropelvic junction (UPJ).Ureteral injuries are graded according to a system developed by AAST. Grade I is a hematoma; grade II is a laceration with <50% transection; grade III is a laceration with >50% transection; grade IV is a complete transection with 2 cm or less of devascularized tissue; and grade V is an avulsion with more than 2 cm of devascularization.

Hematuria is absent in approximately 30% of ureteral injuries. Early clinical indicators of ureteral trauma are vague or nonexistent. Delayed signs or symptoms of a ureteral injury include prolonged ileus, urinary obstruction, urinary leakage, azootemia, fever, persistent flank pain, fistula formation, and eventually sepsis.

Retrograde pyelography is the gold standard for diagnosing ureteral injury, but is often impractical in the trauma patient. CT with delayed images is an acceptable alternative. The most consistent CT finding is extravasation of contrast. On delayed CT images, with a complete ureteral injury there is absence of distal ureteral opacification.

As a result of its tenuous blood supply, even small contusions of the ureter can result in stricture or leak as a result of microvascular damage and should be stented. These patients required ureter stenting for at least 8 weeks in order to allow adequate time for healing.

For more severe injuries, formal repair either at the time of diagnosis or delayed is required. Principles of ureteral repair include: careful mobilization; adequate debridement of nonviable tissue to bleeding edges; spatulated, tension-free, water-tight anastomosis over a stent; use of fine, nonreactive suture; retroperitoneal drainage; and omental interposition wrap when possible.

For lower ureteral injuries, the ureter can usually be reimplanted directly into the bladder in a non-reflux manner, with or without a psoas hitch. A number of other techniques, such as bowel interposition, autotransplant, and Boari flap have been described for bridging longer defects. Alternatively, injuries involving the distal two-thirds of the ureter with insufficient bladder capacity or severe pelvic scarring can be managed by transureteroureterostomy.

References

Alsikafi, N. F., McAninch, J. W., Elliott, S. P. & Garcia, M. (2006). Nonoperative management outcomes of isolated urinary extravasation following renal lacerations due to external trauma. *J. Urol, 176*, 2494-2497.

Altman, A. L., Haas, C., Dinchman, K. H. & Spirnak, J. P. (2000). Selective nonoperative management of blunt grade 5 renal injury. *J Urol, 164*, 27-30, discussion 30-31.

Antoci, J. P. & Schiff, M. J. (1982). Bladder and urethral injuries in patients with pelvic fractures. *J Urol, 128*, 25.

Aragona, F., Pepe, P., Patanè, D., Malfa, P., D'Arrigo, L. & Pennisi, M. (2012). Management of severe blunt renal trauma in adult patients: a 10-year retrospective review from an emergency hospital. *BJU International, 110*, 330-335.

Basta, A. M., Blackmore, C. C. & Wessells, H. (2007). Predicting urethral injury from pelvic fracture patterns in male patients with blunt trauma. *J Urol., 177*, 571-575.

Brandes, S. B. 1. & McAninch, J. W. (1999). Urban free falls and patterns of renal injury: a 20-year experience with 396 cases. *J Trauma, 47*, 643-9.

Brenner, D., Elliston, C., Hall, E. & Berdon, W. (2001). Estimated risks of radiation-induced fatal cancer from pediatric CT. *AJR Am. J. Roentgenol, 176*, 289-296.

Brewer, M. E., Wilmoth, R. J., Enderson, B. L. & Daley, B. J. (2007). Prospective comparison of microscopic and gross hematuria as predictors of bladder injury in blunt trauma. *Urology, 69*, 1086-1089.

Brown, D. F., Rosen, C. L. & Wolfe, R. E. (1997). Renal ultrasonography. *Emerg Med Clin North Am, 15*, 877-893

Brown, S. L., Elder, J. S. & Spirnak, J. P. (1998). Are pediatric patients more susceptible to major renal injury from blunt trauma? A comparative study. *J Urol, 160*, 138–140.

Bruce, L. M., Croce, M. A., Santaniello, J. M., Miller, P. R., Lyden, S. P. & Fabian, T. C. (2001). Blunt renal artery injury: incidence, diagnosis, and management. *Am Surg, 67*, 550-554, discussion 555-556.

Carroll, P. R., McAninch, J. W., Klosterman, P. & Greenblatt, M. (1990). Renovascular trauma: risk assessment, surgical management, and outcome. *J Trauma, 30*, 547-552.

Chandhoke, P. S. & McAninch, J. W. (1998). Detection and significance of microscopic hematuria in patients with blunt renal trauma. *J. Urol, 140*, 16-18.

Chandhoke, P. S. & McAninch, J. W. (1988). Detection and significance of microscopic hematuria in patients with blunt renal trauma. *J Urol, 140*, 16-18.

DiGiacomo, J. C., Rotondo, M. F., Kauder, D. R. & Schwab, C. W. The role of nephrectomy in the acutely injured. *Arch. Surg., 136*, 1045-1049.

Dixon, M. D. (1996). Diagnosis and acutemanagement of posterior urethral disruptions. In: McAninch JW (ed) Traumatic and reconstructive urology. WB Saunders Philadelphia.

Doyle, S. M., Master, V. A. & McAninch, J. W. (2005). Appropriate use of CT in the diagnosis of bladder rupture. *J Am Coll Surg., 200*, 973.

Elliott, S. P. & McAninch, J. W. (2003). Ureteral injuries from external violence: the 25-year experience at San Francisco General Hospital. *J Urol, 170*, 1213-1216.

Gomez, R. G., Ceballos, L., Coburn, M., et al. (2004). Consensus statement on bladder injuries. *BJU Int., 94*, 27-32.

Gonzalez, R. P., Falimirski, M., Holevar, M. R. & Evankovich, C. (1999). Surgical management of renal trauma: is vascular control necessary? *J Trauma, 47*, 1039-1042, discussion 1042-1044.

Hagiwara, A., Sakaki, S., Goto, H., Takenega, K., Fukushima, H., Matuda, H. & Shimazaki, S. (2001). The role of interventional radiology in the management of blunt renal injury: a practical protocol. *J Trauma, 51*, 526-531.

Husmann, D. A., Gilling, P. J., Perry, M. O., Morris, J. S. & Boone, T. B. (1993). Major renal lacerations with a devitalized fragment following blunt abdominal trauma: a comparison between nonoperative (expectant) versus surgical management. *J Urol., 150*, 1774-1777.

Knudson, M. M., Harrison, P. B., Hoyt, D. B., Shatz, D. V., Zietlow, S. P., Bergstein, J. M., Mario, L. A. & McAninch, J. W. (2000). Outcome after major renovascular injuries: a Western trauma association multicenter report. *J Trauma, 49*, 1116-1122.

Koraitim, M. M. (1995). The lessons of 145 posttraumatic posterior urethral strictures treated in 17 years. *J Urol., 153*, 63–55.

Koraitim, M. M. (1996). Pelvic fracture urethral injuries: evaluation of various methods of management. *J Urol., 156*, 1288.

Kotkin, L. & Koch, M. O. (1995). Morbidity associated with nonoperative management of extraperitoneal bladder injuries. *J Trauma, 38*, 895.

Lim, P. H. C. & Chng, H. C. (1989). Initial management of acute urethral injuries. *Br J Urol, 64*, 165.

Matthews, L. A., Smith, E. M. & Spirnak, J. P. (1997). Non-operative treatment of major blunt renal lacerations with urinary extravasation. *J Urol, 157,* 2056–2058.

Mee, S. L., McAninch, J. W., Robinson, A. L., et al. (1989). Radiographic assessment of renal trauma: a 10 year prospective study of patient selection. *J Urol., 141,* 1095–1098.

Meng, M. V. 1., Brandes, S. B. & McAninch, J. W. (1999). Renal trauma: indications and techniques for surgical exploration. *World J Urol., 17,* 71-7.

Miller, K. S. & McAninch, J. W. (1995). Radiographic assessment of renal trauma: our 15 year experience. *J Urol., 154,* 352–355.

Morey, A. F. & McAninch, J. W. (1997). Reconstruction of traumatic posterior urethral strictures. *Tech Urol., 3,* 103–107.

Morey, A. L., McAninch, J. W., Tiller, B. K., et al. (1999). Single shot intraoperative excretory urography for the immediate evaluation of renal trauma. *J Urol., 161,* 1088–1092.

Mouraviev, V. B., Coburn, M. & Santucci, R. A. (2005). The treatment of posterior urethral disruption associated with pelvic fractures: comparative experience of early realignment versus delayed urethroplasty. *J Urol., 173,* 873-876.

Nicolaisen, G. S., McAninch, J. W., Marshall, G. A., et al. (1985). Renal trauma: reevaluation of the indications for radiographic assessment. *J Urol., 133,* 183–186.

Parry, N. G., Rozycki, G. S., Feliciano, D. V., et al. (2002). Traumatic rupture of the urinary bladder: is the suprapubic tube necessary? *J Trauma., 54,* 431–436.

Patterson, B. M. (1995). Pelvic ring injury and associated urologic trauma; an orthopedic perspective. *Semin Urol., 13,* 25.

Perry, M. O. & Husmann, D. A. (1992). Urethral injuries in female. subjects following pelvic fractures. *J Urol., 147,* 139.

Qin, R., Wang, P., Qin, W., Wang, H. & Chen, B. (2002). Diagnosis and treatment of renal trauma in 298 patients. *Chin J Traumatol, 5,* 21-23.

Santucci, R. A. & McAninch, J. W. (2000). Diagnosis and management of renal trauma: past, present and future. *J Am Coll Surg., 191,* 443–451.

Santucci, R. A., McAninch, J. W., Safir, M., Mario, L. A., Service, S. & Segal, M. R. (2001). Validation of the American Association for the Surgery of Trauma organ injury severity scale for the kidney. *J Trauma, 50*(2), 195-200.

Santucci, R. A., Wessells, H., Bartsch, G., et al. (2004). Evaluation and management of renal injuries: consensus statement of the renal trauma subcommittee. *BJU Int., 93,* 937–954.

Toutouzas, K. G., Karaiskakis, M., Kaminski, A. & Velmahos, G. C. (2002). Non-operative management of blunt renal trauma: a prospective study. *Am Surg., 68,* 1097–1103.

Wessells, H., McAninch, J. W. & Meyer, A. (1997). Criteria for management of significant penetrating renal lacerations. *J Urol., 157,* 24–27.

Wessells, H., Morey, A. F. & McAninch, J. W. (1997). Single stage reconstruction of complex anterior urethral strictures: combined tissue transfer techniques. *J Urol., 157,* 1271–1274.

In: Hematuria   ISBN: 978-1-63463-073-3
Editors: Nikhil Vasdev and G. Boustead   © 2015 Nova Science Publishers, Inc.

Chapter 19

Barriers to the Early Diagnosis and Treatment of Haematuria in Secondary Care

James S. A. Green[1,2], Paula Allchorne[3] and Benjamin W. Lamb[1,4]

[1]Department of Urology, Barts Health NHS Trust, London, UK
[2]Department of Health and Social Care, London Southbank University, London, UK
[3]Department of Urology, Guy's and St Thomas' NHS Foundation Trust, London, UK
[4]Department of Surgery and Cancer, Imperial College London, London, UK

Introduction

The Department of Health (DH) Cancer Plans of 2001 and 2003 [1] reiterated the importance of a seamless journey, for all patients with suspected cancer, from primary care to diagnosis and treatment in secondary care. The 2007 Cancer Reform Strategy strengthened these initiatives by defining a timeline in which all patients with cancer must be diagnosed and begin definitive treatment within two months (or 62 days) of being referred to secondary care [2]. The previous chapter looked at barriers in primary care and the important role of the GP in referring the patient. This chapter will look at barriers at the interface of primary and secondary care and those that occur in secondary care.

Barriers and Delays in the Primary- to Secondary-Care Interface

The choice to seek medical advice and which route to take to access secondary care is a personal one but we know that bladder cancer is still discovered in a significant number of patients who present via the emergency route rather than the prescribed fast track 'Two Week Wait' (2WW) referral pathway to a secondary care haematuria clinic. This can affect patient outcomes. Marzouk in a study at a District General Hospital on the outskirts of London in 2011 found that a greater proportion of patients who newly presented to the Emergency Department (ED) with haematuria had a worse prognosis than those who were referred via other pathways. Significantly more patients, who presented via the emergency route, had muscle invasive bladder cancer, had higher grade disease and were older than those referred via the 2WW pathway [3]. The National Cancer Intelligence Network (NCIN) Routes to Diagnosis project reviewed the routes of presentation of cancer patients from 2006-2008 in order to better examine the causative factors in diagnosis delay [4]. This data showed that approximately 19% of newly diagnosed bladder cancers over this time period presented as emergencies. Around a quarter of these (26.5%) were referred by GPs to on-call teams but not to 2 week wait clinics, and 60.7% were referred to the urology service by A&E. The NCIN also found that 12 month relative survival rates varied widely between the two groups with a 36% survival outcome in the emergency group as opposed to 83% in the 2 week wait group. They found that there were higher rates of emergency presentation in the elderly and in those most deprived. In the 50-69 age group, 12% of new diagnoses were made via emergency presentation, compared with 34% in the 85+ age group. Increasing age also had an impact on the 12 month survival in the emergency group with 51% survival in the under 64 group compared to 25% in the over 85 group. Social differences were again apparent in the study population. The likelihood of an emergency presentation with bladder cancer increased with deprivation quintile. It was found that 15% of new cancer diagnoses in the least deprived quintile came through the emergency group compared with 24% in the most deprived quintile. The presentation of older or more deprived patients as emergencies may indicate a failure to access the two week wait system, or it may just be a reflection of the symptoms that accompany the more severe disease seen in the ED sample. Further research is needed to look in depth at the barriers patients may face in accessing the 2WW pathway, and indeed what can be done to improve the timeliness of referrals in general.

An additional concern was that patients when accessing the emergency department (ED) with cancer symptoms, may be experiencing further delays due to the suboptimal onward referral processes. As if the haematuria was not considered sufficiently severe or acute by the ED clinicians, the patient would be referred back to their GP with the advice that a referral to secondary care via the 2WW pathway should be made rather than being fast tracked directly to oncology teams from the ED. This unfortunately had the potential for patients to be "lost" to the system, with 7% of those presenting with frank haematuria to the ED never having their haematuria investigated further [5]. To combat this eventuality the 'Acute Oncology Service' (AOS) was set up nationally to identify patients with cancer related problems who attend the ED, thus providing a means of direct referral to the relevant cancer teams as soon as possible [6]. Haematuria is now one of the defined symptoms that will "trigger" such a fast track referral by the AOS.

Barriers and Delays in Secondary Care

Secondary care delays can be categorized into: first hospital visit; the diagnosis to referral interface, which can involve the MDT; and initiation of definitive treatment. The most obviously delays in secondary care occur from the formation of multiple queues or mini "waiting lists" that are caused by multi-staged processes taking place in a prescribed order. On first look these delays can seem relatively short and inconsequential but when summated they can lead to significant time delays. Some examples of these mini queues involve waiting for common radiological investigations or formalised reports to be dictated, then typed and letters sent. Mini waiting lists or "bottlenecks" can be caused by difficulty accessing scarce resources such as theatres or expensive radiological investigations. There are however other more subtle barriers that are related to other resources that can equally cause barriers and delays. Processes set up with the best intentions can themselves lead to unforeseen delays that may affect patient care. To explore these further we can look at three distinct examples of delay in secondary care within the above categories: 1) one stop clinics, 2) cancer MDT meetings and 3) the 62 day time-to-treatment target.

Appropriate Referral to One-Stop Haematuria Clinics

When patients with haematuria are referred to secondary care via the 2WW pathway they are usually directed to a "one stop clinic" (Chapter 14). This clinic combines components that were previously undertaken separately (an outpatient appointment to take a history, perform an examination and undertake basics tests, radiological imaging of the upper tracts and an outpatient flexible cystoscopy). These component parts occur at one attendance in an attempt to minimise some of the mini waiting lists that multiple appointments can produce. In reality the logistics of this often results in patients spending considerable time in different sites in the hospital. Making sure that these stages occur in the appropriate order and in a timely manner requires significant investment in resources by the healthcare organisation. Barriers and thus delays in secondary care often hinge on the allocation of these resources, which are finite in a socialised system for each financial year. The prioritisation of such resources within a mandatory (government prescribed) time frame can produce unforeseen anomalies, which paradoxically, may adversely affect timely cancer treatment for certain groups of patients. An example of this is the investigation of non-visible haematuria. As mentioned in chapter x, the diagnostic yield (diagnosis of cancer) from investigating non-visible haematuria is less than that of visible haematuria. However, in the UK both usually utilise very similar "one-stop clinic" resources (although slight differences in imaging of the upper tracts do sometimes occur). This anomaly been questioned in recent years with BAUS and the Renal Association publishing a joint consensus statement suggesting that patients who have proteinuria along with non-visible haematuria, may be better served via an alternative route, with referral to renal physicians, thus allowing uro-oncological surgeons to concentrate on those patients with a higher likelihood of malignancy [7]. Unfortunately, as Government guidelines still state that patients with microscopic haematuria should firstly have malignancy excluded, most hospital mangers still persist in using major resources on this group. There is also the added incongruity that the majority of patients who have cancer diagnosed still enter the system via routes other than the standard 2WW referral pathway. In the past only 30% of bladder and 19% of renal cancers were diagnosed via the preferred 2WW route [8]. There is, therefore, a concern that as significant resources are directed to support these one-stop haematuria clinics, 'benign' patient pathways appear to be less of a priority with fewer allocated resources. The fear is that as resources have been redirected to supporting one-stop haematuria clinics, those patients with cancer accessing care through routes such as the ED, and general clinic may now take longer to be diagnosed than before. This is being addressed to some extent with by the Acute Oncology Service (AOS) and by educating GPs to recognise haematuria as a serious symptom and refer accordingly via the 2WW pathway (**see ch x**), but it is still a cause for concern.

Inaccurate Recommendations from MDT Meeting

After a diagnosis of cancer has been made, the most appropriate treatment for the patient must be swiftly decided upon. Others chapters in this book adequately cover the various diagnostic regimes and treatment paradigms for the different diseases that present with the initial symptom of haematuria, but it is important to review the processes involved that lead up to those treatment being undertaken. Many countries now use multidisciplinary team (MDT) meetings or tumour case conferences to aid the clinical decision-making process and optimise treatment outcomes for individual patients. Figure 1 is a schematic model of decision-making in an MDT meeting.

These MDT meeting have been shown to improve chemotherapy regimens and access to radiotherapy [9]. MDT meetings usually they involve cancer surgeons, oncologists, radiologists, pathologists and cancer nurse specialists, with each bringing a different skill set to bear on proceedings. But in order to get the most out of these meetings they have to be well chaired and everybody has to be given "a voice" to state their opinion. Interestingly it has been shown from multiple studies that in up to 15% of cases teams may not reach a treatment decision, and when treatment options are made at such meetings, 4–15% are never implemented [10,11]. This means that a patient is directed down one treatment path only for it to be a "false start" and the patient subsequently has to be redirected down another path. This uses up valuable time and resources.

The commonest reason that most treatment options were never taken up by the patients was usually due to lack of good quality information at the initial discussion. This could be due to poor clinical data (mainly pathological or radiological and co-morbidities than exclude certain treatment choices) but was just as likely to be due to poor quality of the holistic information; family dynamics or support structures, psycho-socials aspect that lead patients to chose one treatment over another. This type of more holistic information is often volunteered by specialist nurses and we found in 6 high performing cancer teams that when these nurses input at meetings was poor they the quality of the holistic and co morbidity information was correspondingly poor (Figure 2) [12].

MDT meetings require a large amount of manpower and time, for preparation and attendance, to function well so it is a waste of time and resources if they do not run as efficiently as possible. If one in seven of case discussions have to be repeated, and one in seven treatment decisions are never implemented, there is a large area of efficiently improvement that can be made and delays averted. Good chairing, good quality information and including all members of the team in the discussion is a good starting point.

TURBT: Diagnostic and Definitive Treatment

The third area to discuss concerns timelines and the perversity that "targets" can sometimes produce. This fact became very apparent during the Mid Staffordshire NHS Foundation Trust Public Inquiry (Francis Report) [13]. But many reports in the press ignored the primary issue. The need to satisfy Government targets led many in senior management in this Trust (clinical and non-clinical) to put theoretical timelines and economic concerns above the clinical priority of patients.

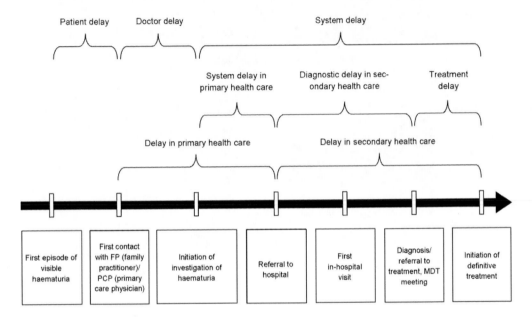

Figure 1. A schematic representation of decision-making in an MDT meeting. This model is based on the input-process-output model of clinical decision-making.

Table 1. One year survival figures for Urological Cancers through different referral routes

Tumour type	One year survival rates by route to diagnosis	
	All	Emergency
Bladder	72%	35%
Kidney	66%	33%
Prostate	95%	54%

Source: 2010. Improving outcomes: a strategy for Cancer [6].

We can sometimes see a milder example of this in the haematuria pathway with regard to transurethral resection of a bladder tumour or tumours (TURBT). As mentioned in the first paragraph of this chapter, in the UK large amounts of resources are devoted to ensure patients get definite treatment in 62 days from primary care referral. This is an honourable aim, but subtle nuances in terminology can change that.

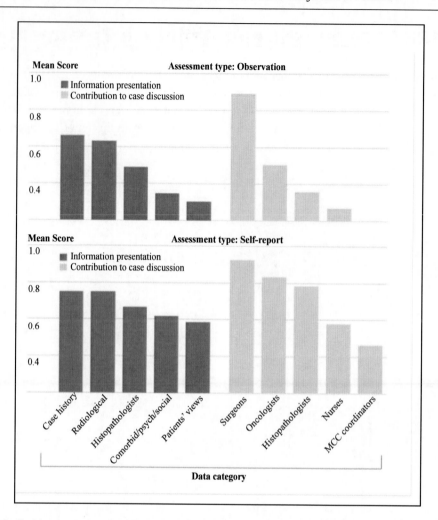

Figure 2. Graphs presenting data from objective observation (top panel) of and self-report (bottom panel) by MDT members on the quality of information presentation and contribution of attendant MDT members (by speciality).

To a cancer manager a TURBT may appear to be a definite treatment, so legally they can "stop the clock", and as the "time line" has been attained Government targets are not breached, and a hefty fine avoided. The commissioners of the service are happy, but that is not the whole truth. A TURBT may be the definitive treatment for low risk superficial tumours, but it is only a diagnostic treatment when the tumour is advanced or muscle invasive [14]. The definitive treatment for this will probably be either a cystectomy or radiotherapy with or without chemotherapy (see ch o and). However, if so many resources have been expended on the initial diagnosis and achievement of this diagnostic TURBT with in the 'target' time, then the resources to speed them that bit further to the definitive treatment may be lacking. The foot has, metaphorically, been taken off the accelerator (or gas). An audit performed in Newcastle exposed the difficulties surrounding this. When clinicians reviewed their bladder cancer pathways for patient with more advanced disease, the time delay following TURBT became apparent [15]. They showed that significant resources were devoted to get the patient speedily to a TURBT, but after this the progress of those with advanced cancer appeared to slow down. Once this had been identified the clinicians laboured hard to find the local resources to take them quickly on to the best definite treatment. TURBT thus needs to be accurately reclassified as both a definitive treatment for superficial bladder cancer but only a diagnostic procedure for more advanced tumours. When TURBT is primarily diagnostic the clock needs to keep ticking in everyone minds (managers and clinicians) and sufficient resources made available until definitive treatment is received.

Conclusion

Hopefully this chapter has given some 'food for thought' to allow those interested in haematuria to look objectively at the patient care pathway [16]. Delays and barriers exist in most healthcare systems and it is important to minimise, and if possible overcome them. It is a challenging task to make patient-centered care as seamless as possible. Negotiating difficult interfaces, whilst at the same time as prioritising precious resources in the most useful areas possible is exceedingly difficult, but never the less important for patient care and increasingly relevant in the current economic environment in which we all practise.

References

[1]   Cancer Plan (2000). Department of Health. (2001 & 2003). *The Cancer Plan*. London: Stationary Office.

[2]   Department of Health. (2007). *Cancer Reform Strategy*. London: Stationary Office.

[3]   Marzouk, S., Lamb, B. W., Harris, A., Mecci, A. J., Gan, J. H., Allchorne, P. & Green, J. S. A. A retrospective cohort study of patients diagnosed with bladder cancer referred with visible haematuria: the impact of source of referral on prognostic indicators

[4]   National Cancer Intelligence Network. Routes to Diagnosis. Public Health England. Available at: http://www.ncin.org.uk/publications/routes_to_diagnosis. Last accessed 18/04/2014.

[5]   see other attachment

[6]   see other attachment

[7]   Anderson, J., Fawcett, D., Feehally, J., et al. (2008). The Renal Association and British Association of Urological Surgeons. Joint Consensus Statement on the Initial Assessment of Haematuria. July.

[8]   Elliss-Brookes, L., McPhail, S., Ives, A., Greenslade, M., Shelton, J., Hiom, S. & Richards. M. (2012). Routes to diagnosis for cancer – determining the patient journey using multiple routine data sets. *Br J Cancer*, October 9, *107*(8), 1220–1226)

[9]   Forrest, L. M., McMillan, D. C., McArdle, C. S. & Dunlop, D. J. (2005). An evaluation of the impact of a multidisciplinary team, in a single centre, on treatment and survival in patients with inoperable non-small-cell lung cancer. *Br J Cancer*, Oct 31, *93*(9), 977-8

[10] Lamb, B. W., Brown, K. F., Nagpal, K., et al. (2011a). Quality of Care Management Decisions by Multidisciplinary Cancer Teams: A Systematic Review. *Ann Surg Oncol.*, *18*, 2116-25.

[11] Lamb, B. W., Sevdalis, N., Benn, J., Vincent, C. & Green, J. S. (2013). Multidisciplinary cancer team meeting structure and treatment decisions: a prospective correlational study. *Ann Surg Oncol.*, *20*(3), 715-22

[12] Lamb, B. W., Sevdalis, N., Mostafid, H., Vincent, C. & Green, J. S. (2011b). Quality improvement in multidisciplinary cancer teams: an investigation of teamwork and clinical decision-making and cross-validation of assessments. *Ann Surg Oncol.*, *18*(13), 3535-43.

[13] The Mid Staffordshire NHS Foundation Trust Public Inquiry. Chaired by Robert Francis QC. Report of the Mid Staffordshire NHS Foundation Trust Public Inquiry. London: The Stationery Office. 2013. Available at http://www.midstaffspublicinquiry. com/report. Last accessed 18/4/14.

[14] Iqbal, S. & Herr, R. (2013). Addressing Delays in the patient pathway for muscle invasive bladder cancer: A National Meeting. Co-chaired by J.S.A.Green and R.Menemim. Manchester. 10th Oct.

[15] James, N. (2013). Do we need to redesign the patient pathway? Addressing Delays in the patient pathway for muscle invasive bladder cancer: A National Meeting. Co-chaired by J.S.A.Green and R.Menemim. Manchester. 10th Oct.

[16] UB40. Food for thought. Graduate Records 1980.

In: Hematuria
Editors: Nikhil Vasdev and G. Boustead

ISBN: 978-1-63463-073-3
© 2015 Nova Science Publishers, Inc.

Chapter 20

The Legal Issues with Misdiagnosis of Hematuria

Kailash Vasdev[1] and Nikhil Vasdev[2]

[1]Senior Advocate, Supreme Court of India
[2]Hertfordshire and South Bedfordshire Robotic Urological Cancer Centre,
Lister Hospital, UK

The practice of medicine devolves on the principles settled by the Hippocratic Oath. It envisages that all medical men "will prescribe regimens for the good of my patients according to my ability and my judgment and *never do harm* to anyone"; "In every house where I come I will enter only for the good of my patients, keeping myself far from all intentional ill-doing" and "All that may come to my knowledge in the exercise of my profession or in daily commerce with men, which ought not to be spread abroad, I will *keep secret* and will never reveal".

It means that every person who enters into the noble profession of medicine undertakes to bring to the exercise of it a reasonable degree of care and skill. This fundamental duty of all medical practitioners has been the cornerstone of ethical practices to be followed and protected by Medical Councils the world over.

In the past complaints of malpractices by doctors were referred to and decided by the Medical Council. With the passage of time with myriad developments in the law being codified, with the rights of individuals being guaranteed by the comity of nations and by individual countries, the right to seek redress in courts brought about an attitudinal change in dealing with cases of medical malpractice and/or negligence. Patients began to take recourse to courts for redemption of alleged wrong caused to them by practitioners of medicine. These are claims in torts upon a breach of a contract.

In contracts the law imposes primary and secondary obligations. A party to a contract must perform what he has undertaken – primary obligation or else pay damages for the consequences to the other party – secondary obligation e.g., a driver of a vehicle on the road must exercise reasonable care and skill (primary obligation) or else pay damages to any person as a result of the driver's negligence (secondary obligation). This principle permeates all cases of negligence and failure to discharge obligations including those in the practice of medicine.

In the United Kingdom medical negligence cases are essentially governed by the principles enunciated by the House of Lords in *Bolam v Friern Hospital Management Committee [1957 – 2 All ER 118] – (Bolam's case) [1]*. The House of Lords in their opinion *held* that a doctor who acts in accordance with a practice accepted as proper by a responsible body of medical men, is not negligent merely because there is a body of opinion that takes a contrary view. Legally, it is settled that in the case of medical man, negligence means failure to act in accordance with the standards of reasonably competent medical men at that time. There may be one or more perfectly proper standards and if he conforms with one of these proper standards, then he is not guilty of negligence. This test now covers the entire field of liability of a doctor in respect of diagnosis *[Maynard v. Midlands Regional Health Authority 1985 [1] ALL ER 635]*, duty to warn his patient of risks inherent in the treatment while holding that English law does not recognise the doctor of informed consent *[Sidaway v. Bethlem Royal Hospital Governors 1985 [1] ALL ER 643]*,: in respect of operating upon or giving medical treatment involving physical force to a patient who is unable to give his consent *[F. v. West Berkshire Health Authority 1989 [2] ALL ER 545]* and liability in respect of treatment giving bonafide.

Treatment by a doctor envisages various positions – standard of care, degree of care, general standards in conduct, confidentiality and responsibility towards a patient. These standards are sacrosanct and binding on all members of the medical fraternity. The Medical Council of Great Britain incorporates these as norms in Guidelines and Rules.

The National Health Service has, to ensure transparency in its functioning set down strict norms in exercise of its power of the earlier National Health Service Act 1977 since replaced by the National Health Service Act of 2006. This Act statutorily recognises by the Secretary of State owes a t duty to provide health care services to patients to such an extent as he considers necessary to meet all reasonable requirements. This is a public law duty and not a direct duty owed to individual patients. The government while emphasising on `Maintaining High Professional Standard In The National Health Service' has set up the National Clinical Assessment Service [NCAS] which operates as a Division of the NHS Litigation Authority. The NHS mandates that apart from following settled guidelines for treatment of patient a `Preserve Confidentiality' policy has been adopted and enforced while handling concern about a doctor's performance. This fiat is an additional safeguard to patients and a breach thereof makes it misconduct for doctors under the trust's disciplinary policy and procedure.

Despite all safeguards and modern gadgets which have brought about radical changes in diagnosis, treatment and surgery, it has not been possible to eliminate negligence in treatment. This becomes a matter of a claim for damages there being a breach of the primary obligations by practicing medical men. Litigation and judicial review of the doctor's actions come into play.

The Courts view medical negligence differently and on a case to case to basis. Negligence by a doctor becomes significant in treatment. This negligence stems from essentially two facets – the failure of a doctor to act reasonably within the norms of settled clinical norms or failure to discharge his obligations as a competent medical man. A totally wrong diagnosis or an incorrect course of surgery comes within the domain of negligence. The failure of a doctor to diagnose an ailment without taking recourse to mandatory norms is unacceptable and necessarily invites action for damages. The negligence in administering a drug or the failure of surgery to exercise reasonable skill and care during an operation e.g., living a swap in the patients for incorrect suturing leading to internal bleeding are acts of negligence. There are myriads instances where courts have awarded damages for acts of negligence where doctors have acted contrary to accepted practice.

Outside the United Kingdom medical negligence is treated differently especially where insurance has been obtained by the patients and by the doctors to protect themselves from malpractice claims. The insurance company invariably seeks to repudiate claims on the smallest pretext. This leads to enormous litigation which involves doctor, the insurer and the hospital. It also opens up a flank for initiating proceedings for cheating against the insurance company for a rash and negligence against the doctor. The consequence is that the doctor's reputation suffers till such time as he is acquitted of the charges. However, pending the trial he has to defend himself against imputations made by both – the claimant and the insurer. In the U.K. where the NHS has its own review system of dealing with patients complaint, the doctor has an opportunity of explaining his position before the National Clinical Assessment Service whose opinion is respected by the courts and of course the Medical Council.

Index

D

F

G

H

Q

R

S

T

U

V

W

Y